BEAUTY BELOW

A GUIDE TO INTIMATE WELLNESS
AND BEAUTY FOR DARK SKIN

By Cynthia M. Wesley, MD, FACOG

*Here's to
Beauty Below!
Dr Cyn*

Published by Swiner Publishing Company

Printed in the United States of America

ISBN: 978-0-578-30113-6

I wrote this book in honor of the female warriors in my life. They infused me with their unconditional love and support. Their displays of courage, resilience, and ingenuity have inspired me to achieve my dreams. I stand proudly on their shoulders:

Mary L. Wesley (the best mom on the planet)

The Late Margaret B. Haley (Granny)

The Late Pastor Mable E. Page

The Late Pearlie S. Page

Shirley Singleton (Auntie)

The Late Janice M. Hampton (Auntie)

The Late Janet F. Johnson (Big Cuz)

The Late Deloris Johnson

Daisy Evans

TABLE OF CONTENTS

Introduction

The beauty market is a multibillion-dollar industry. From our earliest childhood memories, we remember watching commercials, reading print ads, and listening to radio advertisements for various products to take care of our "public" face. On an average day, you will likely see or hear about moisturizers, anti-aging creams, products for zits, and more. But ask yourself: how many times have you ever heard the beauty industry advertise products that protect or improve the skin of our most precious area? Who is teaching us about the skin of the genital area? Of course, we hear about washes that are pH balanced or about anti-itch creams. But is that all the beauty industry has to offer? Over the years, women have taken a more proactive approach to their health and beauty. It's now time for the same attention and effort that is given to our public face to be bestowed upon our most precious Private Face. There should be no confusion about what the Private Face, or our genital area, represents: it's the blossom of a woman.

From the blossom is where we reproduce. So why is such a precious jewel not given more appreciation and attention? In my 20-plus years as a practicing OBGYN, it's clear that many of us just don't know how to give our blossom the attention it needs. We were not properly taught by the women in our families because they were not informed. Unfortunately, society has conditioned many of us to ignore and to be shameful of our unique feminine appearance and needs. After you read this book, your impression and knowledge of the Private Face is bound to change. You should finally be able to know the proper steps to enhance the beauty and maintain the health of the Private Face at every stage of your life.

My first awareness of my vast ignorance of the Private Face was in high school. In my family, we didn't openly talk about "women issues." I can vividly recall my mother and aunts whispering about someone needing a hysterectomy because of something called fibroids. As I perked up my ears to try to catch every word, I remember coming away with the feeling that vaginal bleeding was some horrible thing. A young woman starting her period was like a burden. We weren't even supposed to consider tampons because we were virgins! Imagine that in 2021. I learned that if I couldn't have a frank conversation with the women in my family about bleeding, then I surely was not going to talk to them about grooming my private area. So, where did I receive my elementary pearls for cultivating and priming my Private Face? Well, none other than cheerleading practice.

While wearing a little skirt and only tights underneath, neatness was important. If everyone else was shaving their bikini line, I guessed I had better get to it, too. Needless to say, my first foray into shaving was a nightmare. Initially, the process of shaving was simple enough, but before long, I broke out with itchy bumps. I vowed never to shave my bikini line again. I reverted to using that hair removal cream in the little pink bottle. I was clearly one of the girls wearing short shorts. This method of hair removal was met with some success, so throughout high school on game day, I would pull out the little pink bottle that I kept hidden in my closet. Please recall that this method was met with *some* success. Hair was still there – maybe not as thick, but in random patches. I was embarrassed because I wasn't as neat as my teammates.

After high school, I was fortunate to cheer at a Division I university. This brought added pressure on game day. There was no way I was willing to take a chance at being seen on national television in a perfect heel stretch with pointed toes, straight arms and a wide smile plastered on my face, yet have this shadow looming from my tights. *I think not*. Once again, I went to my teammates. I gave them all the details about my previous experience. After much laughter, I was instructed to shave while in the shower. They were shaving daily using only their shower gel. No one else on the team suffered from bumps. So, off I went to try again. I followed the instructions of my teammates, and everything seemed great. For the first time, I felt confident in my uniform. However, by day 2 of cheering and sweating, my bikini line was on fire! Cool clothes and lotion were not working. *Country roads take me home!* For the next week, I wore oversized sweatpants without underwear. I felt so down, embarrassed, and ashamed. After a full recuperation, I was still left with the task of figuring out a way to groom without it costing me such distress. I realized that the one thing that I was ignoring in my search for answers was that I was asking women for help whose hair was nothing like mine. My hair is coarse, and their hair was fine.

When I looked at my surroundings, I noticed that my dad had the same problem with the hair on his public face. As I started to pay close attention to his grooming techniques, I saw that eventually his solution to his problems came in a black and gold container. It required mixing and stunk to the high heavens. But even with the bad smell, his bumps were gone. I tried the stinky solution on my bikini line, and it worked! As the old saying goes, "You have to take the good with the bad." I started using the solution when my roommate wasn't home, double-bagged the leftovers, and disposed of it outside. A former boyfriend even accused me of cheating because he saw the black and gold container made for men in my cabinet.

Once I became a gynecologist, I realized that many women of all walks of life struggle with figuring out the right way to groom their Private Face. This book will expose you to all your grooming options. It will also help you create the regimen that's best for your skin and hair type. You will learn about solutions and techniques designed for women of all hair types, without the stinky smell.

With over two decades of experience as an OBGYN, I have treated and counseled many women with a host of problems dealing with the Private Face. Some women do not want to remove their genital hair, yet they desire to feel clean, neat, and properly groomed. I've met many women with years of removing their genital hair who suffer from hyper-pigmentation. They are trying to obtain a Private Face that is just as clear and blemish-free as their public face. Some women suffer from sweating in this area. They want and need treatment options. Let's not forget the many women who are new to sex or are returning to sex after a long hiatus. They need to know how to treat the microtears that can occur during "relations" and the daily regimens that are preventative in nature. Over the years, I have developed treatment regimens and products that address these concerns and many more. The many years of labor and love have birthed the Beauty Below Formula. The Beauty Below Formula provides a blueprint to intimate wellness and beauty for dark skin. The formula is broken into four phases. First, you must EMBRACE the Private Face, then KNOW the

Private Face, PAMPER it, and then ultimately OWN the Private Face. I want to share every aspect of my unique approach to intimate wellness and beauty. To accomplish this task, the Beauty Below Formula is divided into two volumes. The book that you are currently reading is Volume 1. In this book, we will cover the first three phases of the Beauty Below Formula. Volume two is reserved for the in-depth exploration of owning the Private Face. All women can benefit from the information provided in this book. As a woman of color, I am fully aware of the lack of acknowledgment of Black skin and its unique expression, especially for the Private Face. This book would be inconsistent with who I am as a Black woman – and as a warrior for all women – if I did not address the physiologic and sociologic factors impacting intimate wellness and beauty of dark skin.

Disclaimer: This book was written for informational purposes only. It is not intended to provide medical advice.

PHASE 1: EMBRACE THE PRIVATE

FACE

CHAPTER 1

BLACK VAGINA CONFIDENCE

ANCIENT CIVILIZATION AND THE PRIVATE FACE

During ancient civilization, the female genitalia and female sexuality were celebrated. This is evident through their statues and stories. The romantic stories of the Egyptian goddess Hathor and her husband, the sun god Ra, talk about how she would show Ra her vulva to brighten his mood when he felt weak.[1] In the Sumerian culture, Inanna is celebrated

---

[1] Graves-Brown, Carolyn (2010). Dancing for Hathor: Women in Ancient Egypt (https://archive.org/

details;DANCINGFORHATHORWOMENINANCI

and worshiped for her sexuality. There are ancient poems that talk about her intimate wetness and fertile fields.[2] The same can be said for the love and respect that is shown to the Yoni, or womb, of the Hindu goddess Shakti. It's hard to pinpoint the exact time in history when female genitalia and female sexuality were associated with negative connotations.

We also know that female sexuality in general didn't garner much respect in ancient Roman and Greek culture. Such negative views are on full display in the story of Messalina. [3] She was the wife of the Roman emperor,

---

ENTEGYPTCAROLYNGRAVVESBROWN/mode/2up). Continuum. ISBN 978-1847250544.

[2] Wolkstein, Diane & Samuel Noah Kramer. (1983). Inanna, Queen of Heaven and Earth: Her Stories and Hymns from Sumer. Harper Perennial.

[3] Anthony Barrett (1996). Agrippina: Sex, Power and Politics in the Early Roman Empire. Yale University Press. Pp. 87, 104.

Claudius. She was seen as a promiscuous seductress with an insatiable desire for sex. She was executed for plotting against her husband. Some historians believe that the campaign against Messalina was politically motivated. As the late Aretha would say, all she was asking for was "just a little respect." Unfortunately, the effects of the negative slant associated with the female genitalia are seen in present-day society. For too many women and men, it is taboo to talk about the Private Face. The female genitalia are seen as dirty. The current landscape has led to women being shameful of the most intimate and powerful part of their body.

HISTORICAL CHALLENGES FOR BLACK WOMEN AND THE PRIVATE FACE

In one way or another, all women have suffered from the disrespectful societal views of the female genitalia and female sexuality. However, it's important to address the unique circumstances that shape the relationship of African

American women and their intimate wellness and beauty. Slavery stripped Black women of control of their own bodies and any sense of security. Enslaved women were raped by their masters and other white men. They were made to procreate with any man selected by their master. The slave woman's body was not her own. In the writings of Dr. Marion Sims, who is considered the godfather of the field of gynecology, he talks about how a slave master loaned him three slave women to use for experimental surgeries. [4] Multiple surgeries were performed without anesthesia.

The negative connotations associated with the female genitalia and sexuality were exacerbated for slave women. They were seen as less than human, ugly, hypersexual with impulse control, tough-skinned, and more. A few years ago, I read an incredible book by Dr. Gail Wyatt entitled *Stolen*

---

[4] Sims J M. On the treatment of vesico-vaginal fistula. American journal of the medical sciences 1852; 23, Jan: 59-87.

Women: Reclaiming Our Sexuality, Taking Back Our Lives.[5]

This book is a must-read. Within the book, Dr. Wyatt breaks down the stereotypes of Black women that were created during slavery. She describes the "she-devil" as a woman who is a cunning seductress that will sleep with any man – even married – without remorse. Dr Wyatt talks about the Mammy, who is seen as asexual, obese, self-sacrificing, and unconcerned about her appearance or overall health. The Mammy stereotype is seen as positive and endearing by both white and black society. Dr. Wyatt also addresses the work horse stereotype. The modern-day work horse is seen as a hard-working, skillful, successful Black woman who comes home to a nice house without a child or a partner. These stereotypes have persisted throughout the years and have impacted societal views of Black female sexuality.

---

[5] Wyatt, G E., Stole Women: Reclaiming Our Sexuality, Taking Back Our Lives; New Jersey: John Wiley & Sons, Inc, 1997.

Due to the conditions of slavery, Black women were not afforded protection or even the feeling of being treasured by the Black men they loved. They were forced to live their lives in survival mode. With the goal of self-protection, Black women disassociated themselves from their own sexuality. The rites of passage into womanhood were no longer shared with the next generation. The Private Face was not discussed, other than to tell the next young girls to keep it covered. Let's not forget that it is still common opinion that the female genitalia are dirty. Black women are conditioned to feel even dirtier than their white counterparts. To combat this notion, Black girls are taught to aggressively clean the Private Face. When it comes to feminine hygiene, the phrase, "Cleanliness is next to godliness," is taken very seriously in the Black community. It's as if the vigorous wiping performed with feminine hygiene will take away all the atrocities against the Black female body. In their efforts to shield themselves and the next generation from the horrors of physical and sexual abuse during slavery, Black women unwittingly wrapped their daughters in the cloth of ignorance and shame.

With all the historical wrongs and current societal pressures, we as Black women have often unknowingly contributed to the shame our sisters feel. Have you ever seen a young Black lady flaunting her sexuality and you gave "that look?" How many times have you referred to another woman of color as fast, hot in the pants, or loose? I know I have. I know I have given "the look" and said, "She's doing too much." Over the years, I've made a conscious effort to correct my wrongs. In my attempts to self-reflect on my behavior to other women, I realized that my actions were a reflex reaction to my own shame. Growing up, I was conditioned to hide or tamp down my natural sensuality. Watching another Black woman show any form of boldness or confidence in her sexuality stirred an insecurity inside of me. The shame I possessed in reference to my Private Face became painfully obvious when I struggled with the simple task of grooming my bikini line. I was mortified when my college boyfriend found the black and gold container of hair removal cream that's made for men under my bathroom sink. His accusations of cheating were easy to refute. The embarrassment and shame came about when I tried to explain why I needed to use the product. It was deeper than an uncomfortable conversation. I was no longer comfortable with his seeing every part of me. I felt ugly and undesirable. I became paranoid about such things as developing an ingrown hair because I knew – with my dark skin – it would leave a mark for at least six months. My shame extended into other aspects of my life. Shame made me feel unworthy of any romantic relationship. The shame became handcuffs around my personality, heart, and even my spirit.

5 STEPS TO EMBRACE THE PRIVATE FACE

Learning to relinquish the shame that I held toward my Private Face was a tedious process. My healing process began in medical school. To be frank, my shame was the catalyst to pursue the field of gynecology. Once I began to truly learn the human body from a medical perspective, I realized that there was a scientific answer to the majority of my problems. I pursued the answers to my problems with a vigor. Even with a wealth of knowledge, I still had yet to embrace my Private Face. I was still suffering and trying to figure out solutions in silence. My patients became my healing balm. As I saw woman after woman with similar struggles as my own, I studied their behavior. I paid attention to their demeanor when I asked sensitive questions. I asked about their familial customs for hygiene regimens. When I would evaluate these women, I saw a reflection of me. My patients gave me the courage and insight to be honest and completely vulnerable with myself. Once I broke the historical chains inside my head and deep inside my heart, I was able to fearlessly examine and appreciate my full nudeness in the mirror, to have conversations with other women about our intimate wellness, and to even have sensitive conversations with my intimate partner. It wasn't until I embraced my Private Face that I was able to have stewardship over my life. It became second nature to say no to any relationship or situation that did not align with my personal goals. My heightened awareness and appreciation of my sensual side amplified my intimate experiences. I stumbled onto the road of female sexuality with medical knowledge as my steering wheel, anger and frustration as my gas, and fear as my brakes. I had no destination in sight. Embracing my Private Face powered the GPS to the final destination of fulfillment and happiness. My new and healthy relationship with my genitalia and sexuality inspired me to help other women embrace their Private Face.

The process of embracing your Private Face does not have to be as long and painful as my journey. The blueprint to the embrace is amazingly straightforward. There is great beauty and power in its simplicity. Here are the five steps to embrace your Private Face:

1. **Look at your Private Face.** It is imperative for every woman to become comfortable looking at her genitalia. You must recognize that vulvas come in many different shapes, colors, and sizes. The appearance of your vulva is unique to you. Look at your Private Face every night with a hand mirror. Look in the mirror every night until you are no longer bothered by what you see. The additional importance of looking in the mirror is to identify any abnormalities. If you are not looking at your Private Face at least once a month, you may miss a medical condition that requires prompt diagnosis and

treatment. Medical conditions of the vulva will be discussed in great detail later in this book.

2. **Say the words, "vulva" and "vagina."** Every morning, for one week, I want you to say the words, "vulva" and "vagina," while looking in the mirror. You must use the terms in proper sentences. Simply saying the words out loud plants the seed to eradicating the stigma associated with the female genitalia. After one week in the mirror, have a conversation about the vulva or vagina with a female friend or family member. Having a conversation with a *group* of women is even better. A great example of a Private Face question is, "Hey ladies, do you ever get ingrown hairs of the vulva? If yes, are there any home remedies that work for you?" Pretty simple, right? You will be amazed at how other women will open up and start talking. So many women have questions, but they're scared to ask for answers even

from their closest friends because of the societal shame placed upon us.

3. **Stop shaming other women.** Sometimes it's hard to break old habits. It may take a while before the reflex thought about another woman being "out there" does not enter your mind. However, you can immediately control the words that come out of our mouth. Catch yourself before speaking anything negative. Then, search your heart as to why you had the thought in the first place.

4. **Have a conversation with your intimate partner about your Private Face.** When you completely embrace your Private Face, there should be no hesitation with having a conversation with your intimate partner about your most precious area. You may discover, for example, that he likes a little hair down there and you've been shaving every other day: damaging your vulvar skin, suffering with ingrown

hairs and the dark spots that come afterwards because you assumed hair removal was something that he desired.

5. **Write a letter to your Private Face.** Here are the questions or topics you should think about and then answer in the letter:

   - What do you like most about your Private Face?

   - What do you dislike about your Private Face?

   - If you could change one thing about your Private Face, what would it be? Why would you want to change it?

   - Name and describe one incident in which you were ashamed of your Private Face.

   - Apologize to your Private Face.

   - Name three reasons why you appreciate your Private Face. Copy your appreciation statements onto a separate index card or sticky note. Place the card beside your bed. Read it every night before you go to bed for one week.

I am confident that any woman can master the embrace of the Private Face if she fully commits to the five-step process. Embracing your intimate wellness and beauty gives you the resolve to tell your own story. With Black vagina confidence, others no longer define who you are. You will boldly and unapologetically let the world know the greatness of your walk, your talk, your passions in life, and even your Black female sexuality. Black vagina confidence is your birthright.

PHASE 2: KNOW THE PRIVATE FACE

CHAPTER 2

BASIC ANATOMY OF THE PRIVATE FACE

Now that you have taken the empowering step of embracing your Private Face, it is time for you to get to know it. In Chapter One, you learned how our ancestors wrapped us in the cloth of ignorance and shame. Ignorance does not mean that you are stupid or unable to learn. Ignorance simply means that you lack information. The dangers of ignorance cannot be underestimated.

Ignorance makes us vulnerable to manipulation by others. The lack of knowledge also increases our risk for delayed diagnosis or misdiagnosis of medical conditions. Now that you have gained the gift of embracing your Private Face, you are able to peel back the shame that has stained the sexuality of Black women. It is now time to wrap yourself and your offspring in a different type of protective cloth called education. By using the weapon of education, you will find freedom in expression, exploration and even love.

Some may feel that the anatomy and function of the Private Face is boring and unnecessary learning. I know differently. *Do not skip the next few chapters.* With true understanding of the Private Face, you will improve your ability to talk openly with the young women in your life, avoid common problems, quickly recognize abnormalities, and effectively communicate any concerns with your healthcare provider.

PARTS OF THE VULVA

In order to truly understand and appreciate the Private Face, it is important to understand the anatomy of the vulva and vaginal opening. Please look at the following diagram as I explain the basic anatomy of this area. As you are learning throughout this book, feel free to refer to the diagram if, at any time, you are unable to visualize the area that is being discussed.

FEMALE EXTERNAL GENITALS

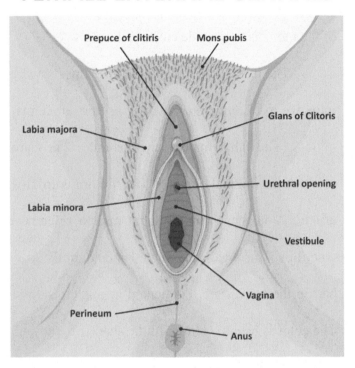

The portion of the vulva that is most commonly noticed is the mons pubis. The mons is the "mound" of fatty tissue or puffy area covering the pelvic bone. In its natural, grown woman state, it is covered with pubic hair. The best way to visualize this area is to imagine standing in front of a full-length mirror with your legs closed. The hairy area that is seen below the belly button is the mons pubis. The function of the mons is to provide cushion during sex.

The labia, which many call the "lips," can be divided into two different areas known as the labia majora and minora. The labia majora are the outer folds around the urethral and vaginal opening. The urethra is from where we urinate. You may hear the labia majora referenced as the outer lips. This area is pigmented and naturally covered with hair in the adult state. Pigmented means the skin has color. The color is usually similar to the shade of your public face. Sometimes the Private Face can be slightly darker or lighter than the public face. If you visually return to your full-length mirror, the labia majora is the hairy area that is seen when you sit on the end of a chair and spread your legs apart. This area starts at the mons pubis. The lower end of the two folds of the labia majora extends in a longitudinal fashion, leading to the anus. The space between the lower portion of the labia majora and the anus is called the perineum. In your imaginary full-length mirror, bend your knees to your chest while in the seated position. This will allow you to see the anus, which is centered right below the labia majora. The perianal area is also hairy. The hair is usually sparse.

The labia minora are the folds that are just inside of the labia majora. These inner lips are not covered with hair. This area is not pigmented. The color of the labia minora is pink. Once again, return to your visualization of the full-length mirror. If you spread the labia majora, you will see the hairless, thin, pink folds of the labia minora. There's no fat here. The function of both the labia majora and minora is to provide coverage to the vaginal and urethral opening. As the top edges of the labia minora come together, they help to form the clitoral hood. If you look in your imaginary mirror and spread apart the labia, you will find a bulge where the folds of the labia minora converge, or come together. Underneath the clitoral hood is the erectile tissue known as the clitoris.

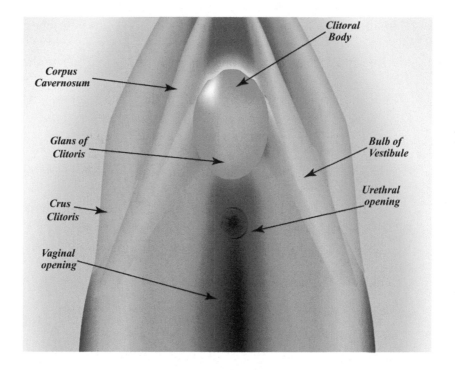

The vestibule of the vagina is basically the porch of a woman's home, or the womb. The bushes around the porch would be the labia minora. This area is noted to begin right below the clitoris. This is the pink area that you see right before entering the vagina. It encompasses the urethra, two different glands, and the vaginal opening. The greater vestibular glands are the Bartholin's gland and the minor vestibular glands are the Skene's glands.

IMPORTANT FUNCTIONS OF THE PRIVATE FACE

- The mons pubis is also called mons Venus or mons Veneris.
- Beneath the labia majora are fatty tissue, blood vessels, nerve endings, and smooth muscle.
- The anus is from where we defecate. The muscles of the anus are the internal and external sphincter. The skin around the anus is looser than the skin of the buttocks. This allows for the dynamic process of defecation to occur without tearing the skin.
- The perianal area is very sensitive, with many nerve endings lying underneath.

- The folds of the labia minora mainly consist of smooth muscles, blood vessels, nerve endings, and some ligaments.

- The clitoral hood is also called the prepuce or foreskin. The clitoris is a highly sensitive area made up of many blood vessels and nerve endings.

- Glands of the vestibule that are immediately below the urethral opening are the Skene's gland. This gland helps to lubricate the urethral opening.

- Along each side of the vestibule, you will find the Bartholin's gland. The Bartholin's gland is the secret weapon that lubricates the vagina.

CHAPTER 3

BASIC CHARACTERISTICS OF THE PRIVATE FACE SKIN

PURPOSE OF THE PRIVATE FACE SKIN

The Private Face skin serves many purposes. One of the main functions is as a barrier. The skin protects the body from external forces and helps to keep bodily fluids inside. The Private Face skin is a rock star with detecting sensation, too. This special area is highly innervated. Other functions of the vulvar skin include thermoregulation and immune responsiveness. The skin contains many blood vessels and active skin appendages, such as hair follicles, sebaceous glands, and sweat glands. Please review the diagram of the skin.

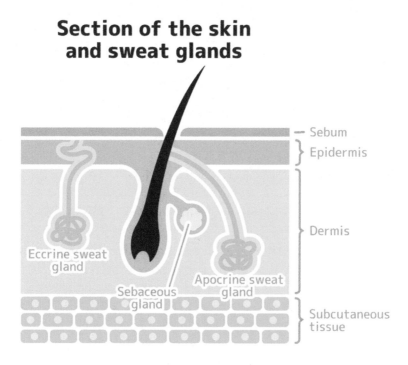

Section of the skin and sweat glands

- Sebum
- Epidermis
- Dermis
- Eccrine sweat gland
- Sebaceous gland
- Apocrine sweat gland
- Subcutaneous tissue

The vulvar skin is made up of three levels: the epidermis, dermis, and subcutaneous level. The epidermis is the top layer of skin. This layer contains a few different cell types, including melanocytes, which produce the melanin – or color – of the skin. The epidermis mainly functions as a barrier. This layer is made up of mostly keratinocytes. These cells produce the tough barrier protein called keratin. Keratinocytes can be viewed as the skin's personal military. They protect the skin from infections, heat, UV radiation and water loss. These cells naturally exfoliate on a daily basis. The middle portion of the skin consists of a layer of connective tissue called the dermis.

The dermis gives the epidermis structural support. You can consider the dermis as the framing of the house and the epidermis as the shingles on the roof. The dermis contains the highway, which transports nutrients and waste from the epidermis. It is mainly composed of collagen and elastic fibers. The collagen provides elasticity and durability. This allows for decreased risk of tearing as a result of sexual relations. The elastic fibers help to maintain normal skin tension. The fibers keep the skin from sagging.

The dermis also consists of an extracellular matrix. You can consider the ground substance to be the sheetrock to your walls. The matrix gives the skin tone. The subcutaneous layer lies below the dermis and contains many fat cells. The functions of the subcutaneous layer are the storage of energy, thermal insulation, and protection from outside forces. This layer provides a cushion when having sex.

The skin of the mons pubis and labia majora is pigmented. In case you're not sure, let's explain pigmentation. Pigmentation is the unique color of your skin. There are three different types of glands of the mons and labia majora: sebaceous, apocrine, and eccrine. The sebaceous glands are the oil-producing glands associated with the hair follicles. The oil that is produced is called sebum. The apocrine and eccrine glands are sweat glands. The sweat glands are usually the culprits that cause the not-so-pleasing smell after exercising or when there is an extended period of time between bathing. The mons pubis is very sensitive to estrogen. As the estrogen increases, the mons pubis continues to grow. The size of the mons pubis can be affected by changes in weight. Many obese women have a large mound for their mons pubis. The perianal region is also considered part of the Private Face. The perianal region includes about a five-centimeter radius around the anal canal. Imagine placing a lime at the opening of the rectum. The area underneath the lime would consist of the perianal region. This area is pigmented with sebaceous and sweat glands.

DIFFERENCES BETWEEN THE PRIVATE FACE AND THE PUBLIC FACE

The Private Face skin is different from the public face skin. The skin down there is slightly thinner than the face that you show every day. Acknowledging that there are slight differences in the skin of the cheeks versus the forehead, the vulva is more transitional than the public face. With the Private Face, there are drastic ranges in skin characteristics. The mons and labia majora are keratinized with hair.

Keratinized means that this area has a lot of proteins called keratin. As previously discussed, cells with keratin are strong and function as a barrier to outside forces. Then there is a gradual change to nonkeratinized, hairless, thinner skin of the labia minora and the vaginal vestibule. The non-keratinized skin easily allows fluid to pass through. Essentially, the Private Face skin transitions from thick to thinner. The thinner skin is more vulnerable to irritants. Compared to the mons pubis, the vaginal vestibule is more permeable, and therefore, more vulnerable to irritants. The vestibule is also more susceptible to friction. The pH of the two faces is slightly different. The public face has a pH ranging from 4.7-5.7. Becoming more acidic, the pH of the vulva is around 4.7. The pH steadily decreases in the vagina. During the reproductive years, the vaginal pH ranges from 3.8-4.5.

You may ask, "Why am I worried about the pH?" Well, the pH determines which organisms, or bugs, can survive in the area. We now understand that when a woman's vaginal pH becomes higher – or more basic – the good bugs die off, and she then becomes more susceptible to infections such as bacterial vaginosis.

ETHNIC DIFFERENCE IN THE VULVAR SKIN

All vulvar skin is not created equally. It is important to know that the skin of the Private Face can show some differences based on ethnicity. The most superficial layer of the epidermis is equally thick in European and African American vulvar skin. However, studies have shown that darker skin is more vulnerable to water loss, thus more vulnerable to drying and irritants. Because of the increased amount of melanin, Black skin develops hyperpigmentation and skin thickening more often. Often, the redness caused by mild irritants goes unnoticed in darker hues. Contact dermatitis, more commonly known as a "breakout," is more commonly noted in white skin.

CHAPTER 4

WHAT MAKES THE PUBIC HAIR SO SPECIAL?

PURPOSE OF THE PUBIC HAIRS

In the modern-day world, many people view pubic hair as a nuisance. However, the hairs down there serve multiple purposes. The pubic hairs function as a barrier to the urethra and vagina from the outside world. They help to keep foreign organisms away. This crop of hair also reduces friction during sex. Each pubic hair is attached to a sebaceous gland which produces sebum. The sebum flows into the pubic hair. Sebum is a natural moisturizer. It keeps the hairs as well as the skin underneath from becoming dry. For those of you removing your pubic hairs, are you replacing the moisture? We will talk about this concept later in the book. Prior to humans wearing clothes, the pubic hairs were seen as a sign of sexual maturity. It is also believed the hairs helped to convey pheromones. Pheromones are chemical substances released from the body that promote sexual attraction from another person. So, if you are removing the hairs, are you making sex more uncomfortable and decreasing your chances of attracting a partner? Just a thought. The other functions include odor-trapping and keeping the skin warm. I can only imagine that this was a very important function many years ago.

TEXTURE, COLOR, AND GROWTH OF THE PUBIC HAIR

The hairs of the Private Face are different than the hairs anywhere else on your body. The hairs are thicker and coarser, regardless of ethnicity. In most people, the hairs down there are curlier than the hair on top of their heads. Some people even have a different color to their pubic hair compared to the rest of the body.

We know that hair in general grows in different phases. There is a growing phase, sleeping phase, and shedding phase. The phases are no different for pubic hairs. The length of growth phase varies from person to person. However, there is a big difference compared to the hair on top of your head. The pubic hairs will only grow to a certain length prior to shedding. Each person's innate length of growth is different. The only other hairs of the body that have this internal stopwatch are the eyelashes.

PUBIC HAIRS AND ETHNICITY

As with the hair on our heads, the Private Face hairs can be quite different based on ethnicity. People of darker hue tend to have thicker, more coarse hair. Their pubic hairs are often curlier. Therefore, people with dark hues are more prone to ingrown hairs. This will be discussed in greater detail later in the book. Thicker and more coarse hair can experience less success with hair removal creams.

PUBIC HAIR CHANGES OVER TIME

The hairs of the private face usually change over time. Women experience thinning of the hairs after entering the postmenopausal phase of life. With the thinning of the hair, those who struggle with ingrown hairs in the reproductive years will usually see a marked decrease in the incidence of ingrown hairs after menopause. And, as the hairs on our heads turn gray, the same process is likely to occur in the pubic region.

CHAPTER 5

BASIC CHARACTERISTICS OF THE VAGINA

FUNCTIONS OF THE VAGINA

The vagina is one of the most dynamic organs of the body. It is a fibromuscular tube that connects the outside world to the inside of a woman's womb. The vagina has two main functions. It imports sperm for potential fertilization of a female egg (ovum). If the fertilization process is successful and pregnancy is produced, then the vagina becomes the export route for vaginal deliveries. Some women question knowing the importance of the basic layers of the vagina. It's important because you must understand the layers to understand how vaginal discharge is produced and to have some baseline understanding of the causes of everyday problems such as vaginal dryness.

LAYERS OF THE VAGINA

Just like the skin of the vulva, the vagina is made up of three layers. However, those layers are markedly different. The vaginal layers are the internal mucosal, the intermediate muscularis, and the external adventitial layer. The internal mucosa is the layer that is in direct contact with the penis at the time of intercourse. These cells are nonkeratinized. There are no mucus secretions or glands in the internal mucosal layer. This layer is not flat, but consists of many peaks and valleys. The internal mucosa contains many elastic fibers and blood vessels. It is also highly innervated.

The intermediate muscularis layer is made up of smooth muscles. The function of these muscles is to expel vaginal and uterine contents by way of contractions. The contractions can range from very mild and unrecognizable to very powerful. For example, the contractions that occur during the pre-menstrual phase are usually unrecognizable.

On the other hand, the contractions that occur during labor are undeniably painful.

The bottom layer of the vagina is the external adventitial layer. This layer helps to provide structural support to the vagina. The large amount of collagen and elastin fibers of the adventitia helps the vagina to expand and adapt to sexual intercourse and childbirth. The external adventitial layer is surrounded by the powerful pelvic floor muscles.

NORMAL VAGINAL DISCHARGE

There are two types of secretions from the vagina. There is basal lubrication, which occurs on a daily basis, and then there is the more pronounced lubrication that occurs with sexual arousal. The capillaries – or small blood vessels – within the internal mucosal layer produce the basal lubrication of the vagina. This lubricant helps to protect the vagina and urethra from infections, as well as provides baseline lubrication to the vaginal tissues to prevent irritation. When a woman becomes sexually aroused, the nervous system enhances the blood flow to the vaginal area and causes engorgement of the venous flow. This process causes the transudate, or discharge, that is noted during sexual arousal and intercourse. The vaginal discharge during sexual arousal is smooth and slippery.

It is normal to have vaginal discharge. Normal vaginal discharge is made up of vaginal skin cells, bacteria, mucus, and the fluid produced by the vagina and cervix. Prior to menopause, women produce about one-half to one teaspoon of vaginal discharge on a daily basis. This discharge is usually clear, slightly cloudy, or white. The discharge can be watery or mucoid. It should not be so heavy that it soaks your panties!

Normal vaginal discharge is essentially odorless. However, the smell of discharge can be affected by multiple factors such as our diet, hydration, and, most importantly, our hygiene habits. Yellow, green, or very thick white discharge is abnormal. It is also abnormal for discharge to have a foul odor or to cause irritation. If any of these symptoms occur, it is imperative for a woman to seek evaluation by a healthcare professional.

VAGINAL PH

You may often hear on commercials promoting a feminine hygiene wash that the particular product is pH balanced for the vagina. You may wonder what the pH has to do with being clean. In Chapter 2, we touched on the fact that the pH controls bad bugs from growing in a particular area. A healthy vagina is acidic, with a pH of 3.8 to 4.5 during the reproductive years. The microflorae are the bacteria or bugs that are naturally found within the vagina. Lactobacillus, a common bacterium, is part of the normal microflora of the vagina. It produces lactic acid. It is the lactic acid that keeps the vagina in an acidic state. The pH of

3.8 to 4.5 prevents harmful bugs from growing in this area. One example of bad bacteria is clue cells. An overgrowth of clue cells can occur when the pH is allowed to rise to a basic level. This process is what causes a common infection called bacterial vaginosis. This is why douching is not recommended. Douching washes away the vagina's good bacteria, which is its normal defense system. There is no need for the vagina to be washed. The vagina is a self-cleaning organ. The natural, daily vaginal discharge removes the internal waste. Therefore, nothing should go inside of the Private Face. It is okay to wash the external surface or the outside portion of the Private Face (the vulva). This area has sweat glands and interacts with outside forces. Not washing the vulva can lead to a bad odor and a build-up of dead skin cells, which can lead to ingrown hairs and/or acne.

CHAPTER 6

PRIVATE FACE CHANGES OVER TIME

As a woman matures, many changes occur throughout her body. The Private Face is no exception: the vulva and vagina change in various ways. It is imperative to teach our young girls about their intimate area. They also need to be comfortable with the appearance. In general, we do a pretty good job with preparing the youth for their first menstrual cycle. Unfortunately, we are dropping the ball in educating them about the potential changes to the appearance of their external genitalia. If young girls were aware that the genital area may darken around the time of their first menses, they would be more accepting of the changes. This is yet another missed opportunity to use the weapon of education to inform young ladies of the natural female process. They are being denied the chance to celebrate this small, but significant step towards womanhood, as opposed to feeling embarrassed by the color changes.

HORMONES AND THE PRIVATE FACE

The primary reason for the changes is the varying concentration of our hormones. Estrogen, progesterone, and testosterone are the hormones that contribute to the transition of the Private Face with age. The most impactful hormone to the dynamic appearance and function of the Private Face is estrogen. This mighty hormone stimulates the production of fat underneath the mons pubis and labia majora. Estrogen is known to increase the thickness of the skin, increase fluid retention, prevent collagen breakdown, and increase swelling of the blood vessels. Thick skin is more resistant to tearing. Keeping fluid within the skin helps to maintain moisture and plumpness of the skin. Preventing collagen breakdown ultimately prevents wrinkles. The increased swelling of blood vessels promotes vaginal lubrication. Estrogen helps to maintain the muscle tone of the pelvis. It also helps to keep the lining of the vagina elastic.

Estrogen can impact the pigmentation of the Private Face. The genitalia of young girls will often darken as they reach puberty. The phenomenon may also be seen with pregnancy. Pregnant women develop hyperpigmentation of the external genitalia. We call this condition melasma gravidarum. The change in color is often more pronounced in women of color. Estrogen also influences the pH of the Private Face. The pH rises in low estrogen states, such as before puberty and menopause. During the reproductive years, our estrogen level is at its peak. During this time, the pH falls, and our vulva and vagina are at its most acidic state.

Progesterone prepares the lining of the uterus to support early pregnancies. It creates a thick bed for the fertilized egg to rest and grow. Progesterone prevents uterine contractions so that the body will not reject the pregnancy. The first part of pregnancy is maintained by progesterone until the placenta takes over nourishing the pregnancy. Unlike estrogen, neither progesterone nor testosterone can directly affect the thickness of the vagina. Testosterone helps to produce estrogen. It contributes to the sex drive of both men and women. Testosterone also increases adrenergic nerve fibers. This means that testosterone improves vaginal stimulation during sex.

MENOPAUSE AND THE PRIVATE FACE

The transition of the Private Face as our estrogen levels decrease is quite impressive. Here is a view of an estrogen-rich environment: during the reproductive years, the vulvar and vaginal thickness are at their highest. With estrogen being steadily available, the mons pubis and labia majora are plump. The skin in this area is toned. The hair of the mons and labia majora is usually thick. Within the vagina, there are multiple lactic acid-producing microbes to help maintain a low, slightly acidic pH. The low pH promotes a healthy vaginal microflora, which helps to prevent infections like bacterial vaginosis. The vaginal lining is thick with multiple folds. The increased blood flow allows for easy lubrication. Due to the high production of elastin, the vagina is pliable and easily stretched to accommodate sex and childbirth.

Now, let's look at an estrogen-poor environment: as women enter the menopausal phase of life, the mons, as well as labia majora, become less prominent secondary to the decrease in the production of collagen. With less production of elastin, wrinkles may also develop. Many women notice a decrease in the thickness and quantity of the pubic hair. As stated earlier, some women may experience graying of the pubic hair. Postmenopausal changes in the vagina produce the most symptoms for the average woman. The vaginal mucosa progressively thins as less estrogen is available. With less collagen, the top layer of the vagina no longer has the peaks and valleys (rugae). With fewer elastin fibers, the vaginal mucosa becomes more prone to tearing. Women become less aroused secondary to a decrease in blood flow to the area. The pH of the vagina increases to a range of between 6.5 to 7.0, secondary to less lactic acid production. Menopause will be discussed in greater detail in Chapter 10.

CHAPTER 7

COMMON PROBLEMS OF THE VULVA

Although the incidence of minor skin problems of the vulva is very high, it is seldom talked about when women are seen for their annual exam. These conditions are not discussed with healthcare providers and are also frowned upon in polite society. Now is the time for you to learn how to prevent and fix these minor but very irritating problems that women have tolerated throughout the ages.

THE SWEAT DOWN THERE

The first problem we are going to discuss is controlling the sweat down there. In general, sweat is important. It is part of the thermoregulation system of the body. As our body temperature rises, sweat cools us down. In addition to being annoying, the sweat down there can cause a host of problems. The most common complication of excessive sweating is odor. The scent can be mild or very strong. Some women become concerned that their partner or even others in close proximity can smell the odor. A chronically warm, moist environment caused by sweating can lead to a breakdown of the skin barrier. A weak barrier can lead to skin irritation and itching. The changes to the skin barrier can increase a woman's risk for local infections, such as yeast or bacterial vaginosis. Unfortunately, some women sweat at the most embarrassing, unexpected times, or they are just sweating too much during activities. As you learned in Chapter 3, there are no sweat glands in the vagina. The vagina is not the problem with this condition. Let's learn the true culprits creating so much sweat on the Private Face.

WHY WE SWEAT DOWN THERE

Pubic hair – One of the biggest problems with sweating down there is pubic hair. As you already know from Chapter 4 pubic hairs function to reduce the friction we may experience from tight clothing and sex, as well as to keep the body warm. The hairs also draw sweat away from the skin. This process can trap bacteria against your skin. The external genitalia have a high concentration of sweat glands – especially apocrine glands – and hair follicles in one place. The unfortunate combination of sweat, sebum produced by the sebaceous glands of your hair follicles, and bacteria can develop a very unflattering smell. The hair can have a bimodal effect on sweating. Since part of the normal pubic hair function is to keep the body warm, a massive garden down there causes women to experience excessive sweating. On the flip side, women without hair can experience excessive sweating, too. The hair is a natural absorbent. It absorbs sweat. If you ever pay attention to the head of a bald man, you will notice that his head sweats a lot quicker and heavier than the person with hair. This is because there's no hair on top of his head to absorb the sweat. The same phenomenon occurs with the Private Face. No hair equals increased sweat. The no-hair situation can occur with natural thinning and less production of hair, as seen with postmenopausal women and with women who choose to remove the hair. If you are experiencing more sweating than you desire on your Private Face, first consider your pubic hair. Is it too much or not enough? Consider finding a happy medium.

Vigorous physical activity – For many women, excessive sweating occurs with exercise. This makes the woman feel uncomfortable.

Excess body weight – Believe it or not, body fat does have beneficial properties. Its main purpose is to serve as the body's natural insulator. Women tend to carry the majority of their weight right around their midsection fat and hips. It's understandable how the fat in these areas can lock in heat and increase sweat on the Private Face.

Tight clothing – Tight clothing insulates heat and therefore increases sweat production.

Non-breathable underwear – Underwear made of nonbreathable material not only traps in the heat, but also does not allow the sweat that is already present to be absorbed.

Pads and panty liners – As with nonbreathable underwear, pads and/or panty liners that are not made of absorbable material will generate heat and not allow the sweat that is produced to be absorbed.

Hyperhidrosis – This is an abnormal amount of excessive sweating unrelated to heat or physical activity. This type of sweating can be quite embarrassing, leading to social anxiety and skin irritation. So how do you know if you have hyperhidrosis? It's best to start with looking for distinguishing features. Has the sweating occurred for at least six months without reason? You may expect to sweat if it's mid-summer in the southern United States, but if you reside in New Jersey and you're sweating year around, you may have hyperhidrosis. Look to see if the sweating is occurring on both sides of the body. Does the sweating disrupt your daily living? Are you experiencing these symptoms at least once a week? If you answered yes to any of these questions, you may have hyperhidrosis.

Hyperhidrosis can be broken down into a primary or secondary condition. Primary hyperhidrosis is usually seen prior to the age of 25, and a family history of the condition is noted. Secondary hyperhidrosis is caused by various medical conditions, such as menopause and hyperthyroidism. Secondary hyperhidrosis can also be a side effect of certain medications. Some anti-depressants such as Nortriptyline and Protriptyline, Pilocarpine, which is used to treat dry mouth, and Zinc, a mineral supplement, may all cause excessive sweating.

PREVENTION OF EXCESS SWEATING

Simple solutions are available to control sweating that is exacerbated with exercise or that occurs when you're doing absolutely nothing.

Private Face hygiene – It is important to wash daily with warm water or a mild soap. While washing, clean within the crevices of the labial folds. Other than daily washing, you also want to wash immediately after exercise.

Thorough drying of the Private Face – After washing, the vulvar area must be completely dried. Secondary to the pubic hairs, sebaceous glands, and sweat glands in this area, the vulvar area is already a warm, moist space. Complete drying prevents excessive sweating and an overgrowth of certain bugs like yeast. Always remember that yeast likes to grow in warm, moist places. Make sure that the towel you're using after bathing is dry itself. You can even use a hairdryer to confirm the complete drying of the Private Face. This is especially true if you are overweight and have difficulty drying between your skin folds. Change out of workout clothing immediately after your exercise is complete. In addition, never leave wet swim bottoms on for an extended period of time.

Loose-fitting clothing – The first thing every woman should do is pay attention to her undergarments. Undergarments that are too tight will cause sweating. Make sure that your undergarments are breathable. Cotton underwear is ideal. Other materials may not be as absorbent as cotton. Furthermore, cotton is a durable, hypoallergenic material.

Avoid Sanitary Pads and Liners – Most sanitary pads and pantiliners are not made of the best absorbable material. If you are using sanitary pads with menstruation, consider an alternate form of protection, if possible. When it comes to sweating, pantiliners can be your friend or your enemy. The liners may become an irritant if they are worn too long. If you need to wear a liner, such as during exercise, please make sure that the liner has absorbable cotton.

Change tampons frequently – It is best to change a tampon every four to six hours. As the tampon reaches its absorbent capacity, the additional blood sits on the skin, which will produce more heat, sweating, and smell.

Powder – Certain powders are okay to use on the vulva. I highly recommend a cornstarch or arrowroot powder base. These powders will help absorb residual sweat, so it's okay to pat a little bit of powder on in the mornings after washing and drying the vulva completely. The powder may also be added prior to vigorous exercise. After exercising, it's important to wash off the old powder. Once the vulva is dried, you may then add a new, thin coat of powder.

Sweat-wicking panties – Sweat-wicking panties are a good option for women with excessive sweating down there and for those who experience increased sweating with exercise. I also recommend sweat-wicking panties for female athletes. They are the ideal underwear for prolonged periods of vigorous training.

Feminine wipes – It is okay to use feminine wipes, especially after exercise. However, do not use wipes that are antibacterial. The antibacterial wipes can destroy our natural defense system and create an environment for bad bacteria to overgrow. After using the feminine wipes, it is best to blot with toilet paper to ensure that the Private Face is thoroughly dry.

Medical treatment – For those with primary or secondary hyperhidrosis, medical-grade treatment is also available. This may consist of aluminum-chloride, hexahydrate sprays such as Drysol, Botox injections, or another class of medications called anticholinergics. The Botox works by interrupting our nervous system's ability to activate our sweat glands. Botox treatment may last for about three to six months. At that point, women will need repeat injections. Anticholinergics work by stopping the sweat glands from activating.

Deodorants – It is not recommended to use deodorant or antiperspirant on your private face. These products may disrupt the pH balance of the vulva and vagina, which may lead to an increased risk for vaginal infections. The products may also be an irritant to the Private Face.

While there are methods to prevent excessive sweating in the private face area, there are times you may also need to seek a medical professional.

When to call the doctor:

- The sweat is accompanied by weight loss
- It mainly occurs at night
- There is fever, shortness of breath, and/or an increased heart rate
- The sweat is accompanied by chest pain, chest pressure, or shortness of breath
- Unexplained sweating greater than six months
- The sweat is accompanied by vaginal discharge and/or itching
- The sweat is accompanied by pain with urination
- The sweat is accompanied by a burning sensation
- There is pain with intercourse

DRYNESS OF THE VULVA

Some women experience dryness of the vulva. Even though vulvar dryness is a common problem experienced by many women, it is seldom discussed. Basic understanding of the function of the skin provides the most necessary tool in combating this irritating problem. The top layer of the skin functions as a barrier. It is made up of dead skin cells and natural oils. Remember from Chapter 4 that the natural oils produced by the skin are called sebum. The sebum contributes to the hydration of the skin and protection from infection. In general, the skin barrier helps to trap moisture, which will keep the skin soft and smooth. If the skin barrier is impaired, and an inadequate amount of water is present, dry skin will develop.

Symptoms of vulvar dryness include itchy or flaky skin, red patches, dull appearance, and rough texture. There are several causes of vulvar dryness. There are also some risk factors, such as family history, increased age, and frequent swimming in chlorinated pools, that could contribute to experiencing vulvar dryness.

CAUSES

Excessive washing – Again, sebum is the natural oil produced by the skin. Too much sebum can lead to acne. In the attempt to prevent acne or an over-concern about cleanliness, too much sebum can be washed away. Too little sebum will lead to dryness of the Private Face.

Harsh chemicals – There are many chemicals found in soaps, cosmetics and even tap water that are damaging to the skin.

Skin disorders – Examples of skin disorders affecting vulvar dryness are seborrheic dermatitis or psoriasis.

Medical conditions – Women who suffer from diabetes, hypothyroidism, malnutrition, Sjogren's syndrome or kidney failure may be more prone to develop vulvar dryness.

Smoking – Not only can smoking cause dry skin, but it also increases your risk of wrinkles, even on the Private Face.

Genetics – Filaggrin is a protein that helps to form and hydrate the skin barrier. About 10 percent of the population has an inherited mutation in the genes that control the production of filaggrin. These people are often diagnosed with eczema at an early age.

Decreased estrogen – As women age, the production of estrogen is decreased. There is less production of the natural oils, which causes the skin barrier to become thinner.

Medications – Acne medications and retinols speed skin cell turnover. Excessive turnover can lead to skin dryness. Also, over-the-counter medications such as antihistamines are known for drying the skin.

Hot water – Hot water disrupts the skin barrier and leads to vulvar dryness. It is best to bathe with lukewarm water. Sure, soaking in tubs for a prolonged period of time can feel very luxurious. I used to soak in the tub until the water turned cold. I would then add more hot water to continue my relaxing bath. Unfortunately, my hands and feet would be wrinkled by the time I exited the tub. I may have felt great after the relaxing bath, but I wasn't being very kind to my Private Face. Yes, it is okay to take a warm, relaxing bath. However, to avoid vulvar dryness, limit your baths to 20 minutes. For those of you who love hot tubs, there are some additional precautions. Avoid public hot tubs and limit your soak time to 15 minutes. Please dry the vulva as soon as you exit the hot tub.

TREATMENT AND PREVENTION OPTIONS FOR VULVAR DRYNESS

In most cases, vulvar dryness is both treatable and preventable. When it comes to treatment, the key is identifying the cause. Often, removing the offending product or behavior is adequate treatment.

Moisturize daily – Moisturizers help to improve the skin's natural barrier. Consider using a moisturizer that is oil-based. Choose an ointment or cream rather than a lotion. These products will help to keep the skin moisturized by promoting water retention. Hyaluronic acid also improves moisture. To help rebuild the skin barrier, look for moisturizers that contain ceramides and lipids.

Use gentle cleansers – Pay attention to the ingredients in your soaps or washes. Try to avoid products that contain sulfates and parabens. Make sure that all your products are alcohol-free. Chapter 14 of this book dives deeper into product selection factors.

Change bathing habits – Avoid hot baths. The water you use to bathe in a tub or in the shower should only be lukewarm. Again, if you choose to take baths often, even though a warm bath can feel soothing, avoid being immersed in the water for an extended period of time. Apply your moisturizer as soon as you exit the water to lock in the moisture.

Exfoliate – Exfoliating helps to remove excess dead skin cells. This will help to smooth out patches on the skin and unclog pores. Avoid over-exfoliation, though. Too much exfoliation can exacerbate the dryness. Consider exfoliating once per week.

Hydrocortisone – Hydrocortisone is a steroid that can be purchased without a prescription in an ointment or cream. The ointment is preferred for vulvar skin dryness. Hydrocortisone helps to reduce swelling, itching and redness that is associated with dry skin.

Estrogen – For menopausal women, the topical application of estrogen can help restore plumpness and moisture of the vulvar skin.

Increase water intake – Eight glasses of water daily are essential to healthy, moisturized, glowing skin of the vulva.

Decrease caffeine intake – If you are drinking more than one caffeinated beverage per day, then you are increasing your risk for dry skin.

Stop smoking – Smoking is the single most negative habit that affects the health of the Private Face.

Avoid hard water – Minerals, such as calcium and magnesium, are found in hard water. They can leave a filmy residue on your skin. The film can lead to skin dryness by preventing moisturizers from being absorbed. Consider adding a water softener to your home water tank or a shower head filter.

Avoid Vitamin A products – In general, Vitamin A helps to regulate the removal of dead skin cells. For those already suffering from dry skin, Vitamin A may exacerbate the problem.

Avoid shaving – Each hair follicle is attached to a sebaceous gland. The gland makes sebum. Sebum is the natural moisturizer for the hair and the skin underneath. When you remove the hair, along with the natural moisturizer, the risk for dry skin is increased.

WHEN TO CALL A DOCTOR:

Most problems with vulvar dryness are due to poor hygiene practices or an over-zealous approach to fixing another problem, like acne. However, there are times when ruling out a more serious problem is a necessity.

If vulvar dryness is not improved with home remedies, it is important to see your doctor. Sleep disturbance is also an indication to make an appointment with a healthcare provider. If open sores or infections develop, I strongly encourage you to schedule an evaluation as soon as possible. If you have a temperature, fever, or chills, your condition is a medical emergency, and you should report to your nearest emergency room.

PAINFUL SEX AND THE VULVA

The fancy name for painful sex is dyspareunia (dis-puh-ROO-nee-uh). The term originates from the early Greek language, meaning "difficulty mating".[6] It is a condition in which a woman experiences persistent or recurrent genital pain associated with sex. The pain can happen just before, during or after intercourse. Dyspareunia is a common phenomenon. About three out of four women experience pain with intercourse at some point during their sexual lifetime. The pain can be felt anywhere in the pelvic region, including the vulva, opening of the vagina (vestibule), vagina, perineum, lower back, uterus, tubes and ovaries (adnexa), or bladder. In this chapter, we will focus on painful sex associated with the vulva.

Pain with intercourse can be very disheartening to a woman. The first step to the resolution of dyspareunia is to assess the characteristics of the pain. Understanding the characteristics of the pain gives you the ability to better voice

---

[6] Agnew A M. (June 1959). "Surgery in the alleviation of dyspareunia". British Medical Journal. 1 (5136): 1510-2.

your symptoms to your healthcare provider. Ask yourself the following questions:

Is the pain primary or secondary?

Primary dyspareunia is pain with intercourse that has existed for a woman's entire sexual lifetime. Secondary dyspareunia occurs after a pain-free period in time.

Is the pain complete or situational?

Complete pain associated with sex means that a woman experiences pain at all times during intercourse. With situational pain, pain only occurs with certain types of stimulation, positions, or partners.

Is the pain superficial or deep?

Superficial pain occurs at the entry, at the time of initial penetration. Deep pain occurs during or after deep penetration.

CAUSES OF VULVAR PAIN WITH SEX

There are a wide range of potential causes for dyspareunia. Based on your answers to the questions above, the source of painful sex can be better identified.

SUPERFICIAL PAIN CAUSES

Injury/irritation – Irritation to the vulva can occur from soaps, shaving, surgery, radiation, or female circumcision.

Skin disorders – Skin disorders, such as eczema, lichen planus or lichen sclerosus, can cause significant superficial dyspareunia. These skin conditions will be discussed further in Chapter 8.

Infection – Infections such as yeast or herpes can lead to pain of the vulva with intercourse. With complicated yeast infections and often with a herpes outbreak, pain with sex can be intolerable.

Vulvodynia (vul-voe-DIN-e-uh) – Vulvodynia is defined as chronic, unexplained pain of the vulva. The pain can be in one location of the vulva or many areas. In addition to sex, the pain can occur with long periods of sitting. Women complain of rawness, soreness, itching, throbbing, and burning of the genital area. The pain is exacerbated with intercourse.

PAINFUL SEX AND YOUR EMOTIONS

Mental illness – Conditions such as anxiety and depression can cause painful sex. Furthermore, some medications used to treat these disorders can negatively affect desire and arousal, which can lead to decreased lubrication and painful intercourse.

Stress – Stress can contribute to the tightening of the pelvic floor muscles, which in turn can cause pain with sex.

Relationship problems – Underlying problems within a relationship, as well as fears of intimacy, can decrease arousal and lead to dyspareunia.

History of sexual abuse – The long-term effects of sexual abuse can be devastating. Even when women are in stable, loving relationships, the previous trauma can lead to dyspareunia within their current relationship.

History of pelvic pain – Women with a history of pelvic pain may develop a fear of intercourse. The fear alone can cause tightening of the pelvic muscles, which can lead to pain.

TREATMENT OPTIONS

Treatment of dyspareunia depends on the cause of the pain. Injuries of the vulva can cause pain with intercourse for a varied period of time. The first step to recovery is pelvic rest. That means no sex. Avoid any further friction to the vulva. During the recovery period, do not exfoliate, shave, wax, sugar, or anything else that might hinder recovery. Continued exposure to friction can worsen the injury, causing infection or scarring.

If you are experiencing vulvar irritation, review the labels on your products. Remove products with fragrance and sulfates. You may also want to consider removing products with parabens. All skin disorders should be evaluated by a doctor.

Any possibility of infection should be immediately evaluated and treated with antibiotics. If you are diagnosed with a sexually transmitted disease (STD), your partner must be made aware of the diagnosis and evaluated. Regardless of which STD is found, make sure that HIV testing is included in your evaluation. Along with antiviral medication, the sores from herpes can be treated with local anesthetics, such as lidocaine ointment, to help relieve the pain.

As discussed before, there is no known cause for vulvodynia. Therefore, there is no true cure for this condition. Treating women with vulvodynia can be complex. In general, treatment is focused on relieving the symptoms. Lidocaine is often used. Your doctor may prescribe antihistamines, tricyclic antidepressants or steroids. Other treatment options include biofeedback therapy, pelvic floor therapy, and sometimes nerve blocks. Please visit the appendix in the back of this book for a list of support groups for women with vulvodynia.

Women with certain skin conditions (discussed in the next chapter), history of previous vulvar surgeries, or radiation therapy are at increased risk for scar tissue. The scar tissue makes the skin less flexible and narrows the opening of the vagina. Imagine the pain some women may suffer with sex. These women may require surgery to remove the scarring and improve their sexual experience.

If there is an emotional component to painful sex, behavioral modifications are helpful. Women can employ a sex therapist to help with their experience. Women with mental illness or a history of abuse should consider a counselor, psychologist, and/or a psychiatrist. Emotional support can be used along with other treatment modalities.

When to see a doctor:

If the pain with intercourse is persistent, it is important to be seen by your doctor. Women also need to be seen if they are experiencing open sores, tears to the skin, fever, chills, or no relief from non-prescription and home remedies. Skin lesions that are causing pain with intercourse may need a biopsy to rule out vulvar cancer.

THE SMELL DOWN THERE AND THE VULVA

What about the smell down there? Is it common to have an odor? Well, a slight odor is very normal. Every woman has a unique smell. You should be evaluated if your smell changes in any way. Many women assume that an abnormal smell down there is coming from the vagina. The vulva is often completely ignored when trying to identify the source of the odor. Well, I'm here to tell you that the vulva may be the culprit. As discussed in Chapter 3 when you were learning about the Private Face, the vulva has the same sweat glands as the ones found in your armpits. We all know how musty the armpits can become without washing them. This is an example of why it's so important to understand the difference between the vulva and the vagina.

I'm sure you all have heard that the vagina is a self-cleaning organ and only water is required for cleaning. I agree with that recommendation. However, many women benefit from hygiene habits that separate the two. I recommend cleaning the vulva with a mild soap or diluted baking soda.

Infection of the hair follicle, called bacterial folliculitis, may also cause a bad odor. Treatment usually consists of an antibacterial wash. Some women may require antibiotics by mouth. Usually, bacterial folliculitis is related to poor hygiene practices or bad grooming techniques. However, women with hidradenitis suppurativa may have a foul odor unrelated to their hygiene practices. We will cover this condition in great detail in Chapter 8.

WHEN TO SEE THE DOCTOR:

If your vulvar odor persists despite good hygiene and home remedies, a visit to your doctor is recommended. You should be seen without delay if you are experiencing fever, chills, swelling, redness, or open sores.

VULVAR ACNE

Just as on your public face, acne can occur on your Private Face. This is yet another reason to give the same care and attention to your vulva as you do the face that receives daily public exposure. Vulvar acne is characterized by inflamed sebaceous glands. As you recall, those are our oil-secreting glands within the hair follicles.

Vulvar acne can be caused by a buildup of dead skin cells and sebum in the hair follicle. The acne may also be caused by contact dermatitis. You are at increased risk for vulvar acne if you experience acne in other areas of the body. Excessive sweating and urinary incontinence can also increase your risk for vulvar acne. The sweat and urine cause a contact dermatitis. Even though they're naturally produced by the body, their prolonged exposure to the vulva causes a breakdown of the skin barrier.

Vulvar acne is a curable situation. There are multiple treatment options that usually do not require a visit to a healthcare provider. Many women benefit from warm compresses or sitz baths, controlling vulvar sweat, and/or avoiding irritating agents. For contact dermatitis, it can become difficult to identify the offending agent. Confirm if you changed bubble baths, detergents, or other products within the past month. Others may require the use of benzoyl peroxide. If benzoyl peroxide is used, I recommend a concentration of five percent or less. If the pain or skin darkening associated with vulvar acne is severe, your doctor may provide steroid injections to control the inflammation that is causing the symptoms.

PREVENTATIVE MEASURES

KEEP THE VULVA DRY! – I see so many women with vulvar acne who leave the gym in the same yoga pants worn for their extensive workout. They go to the grocery store, stop at the gas station, take the dog for a walk, and talk to their girlfriends on the phone prior to showering. That is the perfect setup for acne. Those little bugs are having a party in that warm, moist environment. The same is true for women who hang out at the pool in their swimsuit bottoms for the entire day. After exercising or swimming, wash the vulva and replace your wet clothes with something dry and cotton.

Avoid tight clothing – I cannot say this enough. Tight clothing is not your friend. If the undergarments or pants are too tight, it increases your risk of sweating, creates a buildup of dead skin cells and sebum, and increases the friction down there, which can disrupt the skin barrier.

Exfoliate – Exfoliate, especially if you are a woman who removes the pubic hairs.

Use a mild wash – The pH of some soaps can be quite high. The high pH can disrupt the natural flora of the vulva.

Use a special razor – If you are shaving, only use the razor for your Private Face. I often remind women to use a special razor on their special area. Having a razor specifically for the Private Face will decrease the chance for infection. It will also help to ensure that the razor remains sharp.

Do not pick or pop a bump – This can damage the skin and spread infection.

WHEN TO CALL THE DOCTOR:

In general, vulvar acne is a common problem that is not a medical emergency. However, there are times when a proper evaluation by a healthcare provider can identify an underlying problem or prevent worsening of this condition. It's important to see a doctor if your symptoms are not improving. If you develop increased pain, fever/chills, and/or swollen lymph nodes, a visit to the doctor is imperative. Anytime you experience abnormal vaginal bleeding or discharge, a proper evaluation by a healthcare provider is highly recommended.

INGROWN HAIRS

Many women suffer from ingrown hairs. First, let's make sure we understand what constitutes ingrown hair. Normally, the hair grows straight up like a blade of grass. An ingrown hair is a benign condition that occurs when the hair curls back upon itself and into the hair follicle, or pierces the skin beside the hair follicle and grows underneath. Please review the following diagram:

INGROWN HAIRS

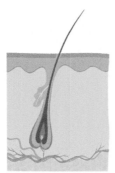

The normal state of the hair

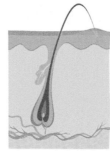

Hair has grown back on itself and back into the skin surface

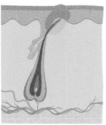

Hair has blocked from growing out and started to grow to the side

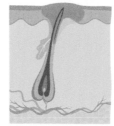

Hair is trapped on it's way out of the skin

There are two types of ingrown hair conditions: extrafollicular penetration and trans follicular penetration. An extrafollicular penetration ingrown hair occurs when the hair follicle curls around, pierces the skin, and grows next to the hair follicle. It is commonly seen with shaving. When hair is removed with shaving, a sharp tip is left. It is the sharp tip that can penetrate the skin when it curves around. The second type of ingrown hair is called trans follicular penetration. This type of ingrown hair is commonly seen with tweezing. With tweezing, a part of the hair is left inside of the hair follicle. As that piece of hair starts to grow, it is unable to move upward through the follicle. Therefore, it grows through the follicle walls and into the skin next to the follicle.

CAUSES OF INGROWN HAIR

The most talked-about cause of ingrown hairs is shaving. Once again, when the hair is shaved, it is broken in an uneven fashion, causing a sharp tip. That sharp tip has the ability to pierce the skin as it curls around. Although to a lesser extent, this process can also occur with waxing and sugaring.

However, not all ingrown hairs are caused by mechanical manipulation. Some people, especially those who have coarse or curly hair, may develop ingrown hairs even without shaving. Research has also shown that there is a genetic component to ingrown hairs in which there are changes to the gene expression of keratin, which is the main protein that makes up the structure of hair. The ingrown hairs can also be caused by a lack of natural exfoliation of the skin. The skin can clog the hair follicle. A clogged hair follicle forces the hair to grow sideways under the skin. This is the same situation that can occur with tweezing.

SYMPTOMS

Hair is meant to grow inside of dedicated channels.

These channels are our hair follicles. Once hair is growing inside of the body but outside of the hair follicle – either from extrafollicular penetration or trans follicular penetration – the body sees the hair as a foreign body. The body will attack any foreign body. The body's attack on the hair causes an inflammatory reaction. The inflammatory reaction causes the symptoms that are commonly seen with ingrown hair. The common symptoms are the following:

- Flesh-colored or red bumps that are also called papules (look like pimples)
- Boil-like sores filled with pus that are also called pustules
- Erythema, or redness, around the follicle
- Pain
- Itching

RISK FACTORS

In the majority of cases, ingrown hairs are completely preventable. For most women, simply stopping shaving, waxing, or sugaring is the answer. For others, prevention is a more complex process and not always 100-percent possible. The following list includes risk factors for ingrown hairs:

Hair removal – As stated before, with most hair removal techniques, the shaft of the hair is cut at an angle. The tip of the angle can pierce the skin and grow underneath. This process is more likely with shaving. It is less likely with waxing and sugaring, but still possible.

Increased sex hormones – Women with certain conditions such as Polycystic Ovarian Syndrome (PCOS), Congenital Adrenal Hyperplasia, or Hirsutism will have increased levels of sex hormones such as testosterone. This leads to an overgrowth of unwanted body hair.

Brittle hair and dry skin – Brittle hair easily breaks and can lead to sharp tips that easily penetrate the skin. Dry skin often has many layers of dead skin, which clog the hair follicles. This is often seen in women with conditions of the thyroid.

Thick, coarse, and/or curly hair – Hair structure and direction of growth play an important role in whether a person will experience ingrown hairs. Course or curly hair is more likely to bend back and re-enter the skin. This is especially true in people with these hair types who choose to shave or cut the hair. There is a particular type of ingrown hair, pseudo-folliculitis barbae, that is commonly seen in people of color. We will address this condition separately.

PSEUDO-FOLLICULITIS BARBAE

Pseudo-folliculitis barbae is also known as razor bumps. With this condition, there is inflammation of the hair follicles without infection. The condition is often seen in people of African descent because of the curvature of the African hair follicle. The condition can occur without removing hair but is more likely to occur after shaving, waxing, sugaring, or tweezing. This condition was first noted in men, which is why it was given the name pseudo-folliculitis barbae. Men commonly develop these razor bumps shortly after shaving.

Flesh-colored or red bumps with the hair shaft in the center are seen in shaved areas next to the hair follicle opening. These bumps can sometimes turn into pustules or abscesses from bacteria on the skin. Due to the inflammation stimulating the melanocytes, which produce melanin, more pigmentation is produced, which leads to post-inflammatory hyperpigmentation of the skin. People can also develop scarring and, rarely, keloid formation. Although it was first noted and commonly seen in the beard area, women can develop this condition in their pubic region. Much attention must be given to people with the chronic condition of pseudo-folliculitis barbae when it comes to treatment and prevention.

COMPLICATIONS

- Infection – bacterial folliculitis
- Hyperpigmentation – darkening of the skin
- Scarring – sometimes Keloid formation

TREATMENT

Ingrown hairs commonly resolve on their own without any intervention. The most important part of the healing process is keeping the area clean. There are many bacteria on the surface of the skin. It is important to keep bacteria from entering the area involved. One must avoid shaving during the time of having ingrown hair. Shaving will only cause increased irritation and inflammation. Picking the area or trying to tweeze the area will cause more harm than good and increase the risk for bacterial infection. However, if the ingrown hair is visible and a portion of it is not under the skin, it *is* okay to tweeze the hair.

It is so hard to avoid the temptation of popping a cyst, but you must not do so. The yellow substance released from the cyst is keratin. If you bust a cyst and release the yellow fluid, the cyst wall will still be present, which allows the cyst to regrow. Popping a cyst can also introduce bacteria from the skin into the cyst, causing either a bacterial infection and/or a bigger, more painful bump.

Rather than re-shaving or popping a cyst to try to cure ingrown hairs, here is a list of treatment options:

- Warm Compress – Apply for 10-15 minutes at least three times per day.

- Antiseptic Solution – An example is tea tree oil, which will soothe the itch and pain.

- Exfoliation – Continued exfoliation with a mild product

- Over-the-counter (OTC) Triple Antibiotic Ointment

- OTC Benzoyl Peroxide

- OTC Steroid – Hydrocortisone, for example, will ease the swelling and irritation

- Topical Prescription Antibiotics

- Oral Prescription Antibiotics

- Retinoids (Retin-A) – Removes dead skin cells and reduces skin pigment changes

PREVENTION TECHNIQUES:

Ingrown hairs are a nagging and uncomfortable problem to deal with. Even though they are benign, they can lead to much discomfort, bacterial infections, and darkening – or even scarring – of the skin. That is why it's important for us to do all we can to prevent ingrown hairs. Here is a list of various techniques to prevent ingrown hairs:

Stop removing your pubic hairs – For most people, leaving the pubic hairs in place will solve the issue of ingrown hairs. Pubic hair removal does not improve hygiene. Therefore, there is no real reason to remove it. One can simply trim the area for an aesthetically pleasing effect.

Use other hair removal techniques – If removing the hairs from your Private Face is an absolute necessity, please avoid shaving, waxing, sugaring, or tweezing. Other hair removal options include:

Depilatory creams – The protein of the hair is called keratin. These creams dissolve the protein at the base of the hair so that it can be easily removed from the skin when wiping the cream away. These products are usually applied to the unwanted hair for 5-10 minutes and then wiped away with a warm cloth. It is important to test a small area of skin prior to overall use. The chemicals in depilatory creams are strong, and people may develop a reaction. Your hair will grow back pretty quickly.

Laser hair removal – Laser hair removal works by emitting a concentrated beam of light through the skin to selectively damage the hair follicles. By stunning the hair follicles, the beam inhibits or delays future hair growth. This technique will not work on very blonde, white, or gray hair. The light is absorbed by the melanin in the hair, so laser hair removal works best on dark hair. This procedure is fast and efficient but usually requires more than one treatment. Laser hair removal can cause some skin discoloration.

Electrolysis – This procedure can be performed on any color of skin and any thickness or color of hair. With this procedure, a needle is inserted into the skin, and an electrical current targets individual hair follicles. The current heats the area around the hair follicle, which damages the follicle and causes it to break. The hair will then fall out. This procedure leads to permanent hair removal. The downside is that it is a very slow and tedious process. It requires multiple treatments.

Loose clothing – Loose clothing does not fit snuggly to the body. It is not restrictive, allowing the body, especially the Private Face, to breathe. There is less friction to the skin and hair follicles, which decreases the likelihood of clogging the hair follicles.

Exfoliation – Other than not removing the pubic hairs, exfoliation is one of the best things you can do to prevent ingrown hairs. Exfoliation helps to remove dead skin cells. It also helps to catch those hairs that are bending back and just entering the skin to release them. This process can be accomplished in many ways. If you are someone with a full garden, meaning that you keep greater than 50 percent of the hair down there (we will talk about this more toward the end of the book), you can accomplish exfoliation by using a thin tooth comb while in the shower. This will help to remove dead skin cells and catch those hairs before they dive in too deeply. For those with less hair or no hair on the Private Face, you can exfoliate by other methods. One method is by using a dry brush. This can be used prior to entering the shower. Not only will it remove dead skin and catch little hairs, but it will also stimulate your lymphatic system to remove toxins from your body. A soft-bristled toothbrush can also be used for the Private Face. One may also use a mild, gentle scrub or solutions that are made for exfoliation.

Stop tweezing – I believe this option speaks for itself. Again, with tweezing, a portion of the hair can be left down inside of the hair follicle. If this hair has trouble getting out, it can grow through the wall of the follicle and therefore cause ingrown hair.

Hair softener – For those of you with a full garden who are prone to ingrown hairs, I recommend a hair softener. Hair softeners are commonly used on beards. A hair softener keeps the tips of the hair from being sharp, and therefore when a follicle curves around, it will hopefully be unable to penetrate the skin. This will prevent ingrown hairs.

Moisturize the skin – it is important to make sure that the skin is not dry. Healthy moisture of the skin prevents the buildup of dead skin cells and will also contribute to softening the pubic hairs. This is especially important to those of you who are removing your pubic hair.

Incorporate proper shaving techniques – If it is imperative that you shave, proper shaving techniques are a must. Here are some tried and true techniques:

- Wash with warm water or a mild cleanser prior to shaving.

- Exfoliate prior to shaving.

- Use a shave gel or shave cream. This will help to soften the hairs.

- Use a sharp, single-blade razor. If you are using disposable razors, only use them three times and then switch.

- Use a special razor for your special area. Do not use the same razor for the Private Face that you use for your armpits and legs.

- Shave in the same direction as hair growth. Shaving in the opposite direction will cause a sharp break in the hair and thus increase your risk for ingrown hairs.

- Do not shave too close to the skin.

- Limit the strokes of the razor.

- Rinse the blade with water after each stroke.

- Do not pull the skin too tight when shaving. Pulling the skin tightly allows the hair to re-enter the follicle without first growing out.

- Use an aftershave solution. This helps to rehydrate the skin.

- Hold electric razors slightly above the skin when shaving.

WHEN TO SEE THE DOCTOR:

Knowing when to seek professional help is very important. Waiting too late can sometimes have permanent consequences. If the ingrown hairs do not clear up within one week, a trip to the doctor is warranted. If the ingrown hairs are causing worsening pain and/or drainage, a medical evaluation is recommended. An immediate appointment should be made if the ingrown hairs show spreading of the reddened area or if you are experiencing fever and/or chills. Women with uncontrolled diabetes or a weakened immune system, such as with HIV, should seek care if they have worsening bumps.

HYPERPIGMENTATION

Hyperpigmentation is an area of the skin that is darker relative to the lighter skin around it. This phenomenon most commonly occurs when the melanocytes are stimulated to produce more melanin. The additional melanin causes more pigment to be deposited on the skin. Hyperpigmentation can also be present when the pigment is deposited deep within the skin, resulting in dark spots. This usually occurs secondary to an inflammatory process. It is the inflammation that stimulates melanin production. People with darker skin are more prone to the development of hyperpigmentation. The pigment cells (melanocytes) are more reactive and prone to discoloration in people of color. Even though this is a harmless condition for some, the hyperpigmented skin can take up to two years to resolve. Many women find discomfort in having dark areas on their Private Face.

The over-production of melanin with hyperpigmentation can be triggered by the sun, hormonal changes, and inflammation/trauma. Due to the location, the sun plays an insignificant role in skin darkening on the Private Face. Pigment cells in the genital area are very sensitive to hormones. When women experience a surge of estrogen, such as during the time of puberty or pregnancy, dark patches of skin may occur. The darkening of the genitalia that begins with puberty never goes away. For many women – especially women of color – the darkening continues with age. Melasma gravidarum is the hormonally driven development of dark patches during pregnancy. Many people refer to this condition as the mask of pregnancy. It is

117

most commonly seen on the cheek bones, forehead, upper lip, nose, and lateral neck. Melasma can also occur in other areas, including the Private Face. There may be a genetic component related to the tendencies of developing melasma. Melasma is more common in Black women. Hormone-related hyperpigmentation may also develop secondary to birth control pills or certain medical conditions, such as diabetes, hyperthyroidism, or Addison's disease.

Post-inflammatory hyperpigmentation (PIH) is the most common type of skin darkening that affects the Private Face. PIH generally occurs in response to injury of the skin. The injury of the skin causes inflammation, which stimulates the skin to over-produce melanin. The increased melanin results in discoloration and an uneven skin tone. It can occur regardless of skin color. However, the darker the skin, the more likely that person can develop PIH. It is common and normal for women to notice darkening of the skin at the inner thighs or in the anogenital area. The darkening has likely occurred over time because of friction. Often, PIH is seen in intertriginous areas. This simply means where two different areas of skin rub together. If you think about it, our thighs are likely rubbing together and creating friction every time we're walking. Hyperpigmentation can also occur with vulvar acne or ingrown hairs. Due to the increased propensity for the development of PIH, women of color should be aggressive with early treatment of acne and/or ingrown hairs.

TREATMENT OPTIONS:

There is no true medical complication from hyperpigmentation. Therefore, treatment is really related to cosmetic concerns. The first line of treatment is the removal of the offending agent and/or treatment of the underlying condition. If you noticed hyperpigmentation after starting birth control pills, talk to your healthcare provider about other contraceptive options. If you are developing post-inflammatory hyperpigmentation with shaving, please stop shaving, or, at a minimum, re-evaluate your shaving technique and pre- and post- shaving regimen. Patience is the simplest form of treatment, but the hardest for compliance. If the offending agents are removed, many women experience spontaneous resolution of hyperpigmentation. On the other hand, some women, especially women of color, can experience delayed recovery. The dark spot can take years to fade away.

Multiple home remedies have been touted to improve hyperpigmentation. It's important to note that there is little scientific evidence to support these claims. Most natural remedies are unlikely to cause harm. In my opinion, they are worth trying. Lemon juice and tea tree oil has been used for many years as a skin brightener. I do not recommend their use in a pure form for hyperpigmentation of the Private Face. They have been shown to cause irritation. Increased irritation may worsen your hyperpigmentation. Adding a few drops of lemon juice to a baking soda paste will be less likely to cause irritation. Other natural products to consider are aloe vera gel, turmeric, green tea, or papayas. Look for products that contain licorice root extract, bear berry extract, or azelaic amino acid. Vitamin C is mainly known for its antioxidant properties. However, Vitamin C also decreases the formation of melanin and increases collagen formation. Pure Vitamin C, L-ascorbic acid, can be very harsh and irritating. I do not recommend L-ascorbic acid for the Private Face. A Vitamin C derivative, such as magnesium ascorbyl phosphate, is better suited for the genital area.

There are advanced options for the treatment of hyperpigmentation of the Private Face. Over-the-counter (OTC) and prescription strength medications, such as hydroquinone, kojic acid, and retinoids, can be used to treat hyperpigmentation. Even with OTC options, the use of these medications for the Private Face should be done with caution. Chemical peels can be used to treat hyperpigmentation. They provide a deep exfoliation of the skin. Both microdermabrasion and micro-needling are effective for hyperpigmentation. Various lasers are also beneficial for the treatment of hyperpigmentation. Advanced treatment options will be discussed in great detail in Volume 2 of *Beauty Below*.

CHAPTER 8

MEDICAL PROBLEMS OF THE VULVA

Just as any other area of the body, various medical problems may present themselves on the vulvar skin. Now, solutions to medical conditions of the skin should not be handled as a Do-It-Yourself project. Initial treatment options and maintenance may include home remedies or over-the-counter medication. However, early medical evaluation is important. With most of these conditions, delay in diagnosis and treatment can lead to long-term or even permanent damage to the skin of the vulva. We also want to make sure that we never miss a cancerous lesion. In this chapter, we will dive into the background of the most common medical conditions of the vulvar skin.

STDs AND THE VULVA

Many people only think of the vagina when

considering sexually transmitted diseases. However, some STDs also affect the vulva. The most common example is genital herpes. Some women with herpes may not have any symptoms. Others will likely present with a very tender, blister-like sore on the external genitalia. Some women may have flu-like symptoms with their first outbreak. There may be more than one blister. It is easy to confuse a herpes lesion with other skin conditions, such as an ingrown hair. I recommend evaluation by a healthcare provider for any new, painful lesion on the Private Face. Herpes can be transmitted by coming in contact with a herpes sore, saliva, and skin of the mouth or genitals even when the infected person does not have symptoms. Although herpes is relatively easy to spread, you will not contract herpes from a towel, swimming pool or toilet seat. It is important to note that there is not cure for herpes and the frequency of outbreaks vary from person to person. Herpes is treated with antiviral medications. Early treatment and suppressive therapy can decrease the frequency of recurrence. Please inform your partner if you are diagnosed with herpes. Proper genital hygiene during a herpes outbreak can improve our quality of life. Avoid sex and any other forms of friction during an outbreak and until the lesion is completely healed. Do not touch the sores. Wash with a mild soap and pat dry. Wash your hands thoroughly. Do not touch your eyes when you have an outbreak. A lidocaine ointment can help with the pain associated with the sores. Along with loose clothing during the day, consider going without underwear at night. Often, the diagnosis of herpes can lead to emotional distress. If you fall into this category, please visit the appendix in the back of this book for a list of support groups.

Syphilis is another sexually transmitted disease that can affect the vulva. Unlike the painful sores seen with herpes, syphilis initially shows up as a non-tender, firm, round sore of the genitalia. This STD can cause serious health problems if untreated. Early treatment is a must. Some women may develop a rash, swollen lymph nodes and fever. The third stage of syphilis can cause serious medical problems. Women can develop serious conditions of the heart, brain, and other organs. On a positive note, syphilis can be cured. I cannot stress this enough: if you are unsure of the cause of any bump or sore on the Private Face, please see your doctor.

LICHEN SIMPLEX CHRONICUS

Vulvar lichen simplex chronicus is essentially chronic eczema. Eczema is a skin condition that makes the skin dry, itchy and sometimes inflamed. In this condition, the vulvar skin develops thick, leathery, scaly areas. These areas cause intense itching. The thickness of the skin occurs secondary to chronic itching and scratching. For many women, the itching disrupts their sleep. Other than chronic irritation, the true cause of lichen sclerosis chronicus is unknown. It is believed that genetics, improper functioning of the immune system and an abnormality in the protein that maintains the membrane of the skin cells may all play a role in the cause of lichen simplex chronicus. The age of onset for this condition is usually mid- to late adulthood. Lichen simplex chronicus is diagnosed by biopsy.

For most women with lichen simplex chronicus, the skin will show a rash that appears red and dry. For women of color, lichen simplex chronicus can look quite different. Black skin may look dark brown, purple or an ashen gray color. Women of color have more severe forms of lichen simplex chronicus with extensive dryness. After flares, black skin may appear darker or lighter (hyperpigmentation or hypopigmentation). Unique to women of color is papular eczema. This eczema appears as multiple, dark bumps that look like goose bumps. When papular eczema develops around the hair follicles, it's called follicular accentuation. Often, it's hard to see a rash in dark skin. With the difficulty in identifying a rash and the varied presentations of lichen simplex chronicus, women of color are often misdiagnosed. The delay in treatment can lead to pigmented changes, such as hyper and hypopigmentation.

There is no cure for lichen simplex chronicus. Therefore, it is imperative for women to pay close attention to their hygiene habits. In Chapter 12, I discuss healthy hygiene habits in detail. Proper treatment options should be started as soon as the return of itching or burning occurs. Improper treatment can often make the condition worse. First, women need to make note of their hygiene habits, including washing techniques, all soaps, creams, laundry detergents, and other products. Anything that comes in contact with your Private Face, write it down. Give this information to your healthcare provider. Your provider should make sure that a contact dermatitis is not at the root of your problem. Some may even require a patch test, which looks for specific allergens (substances that are causing you to itch). If an irritant is found, it can easily be removed from your hygiene habits. Soaking in warm baths and patting dry can help relieve the itch. The water also helps to hydrate the skin. In patients with lichen simplex chronicus, the baths should be limited to no longer than 10 minutes. During a flare, moisturizing the vulva at least twice a day is essential to relief. Topical steroids are the gold standard for treatment. Topical, low dose steroids are applied to the skin for a limited time frame and no more than twice per day. Tar extract (without alcohol) and antihistamines may also be recommended by our doctor. If the symptoms are severe, your doctor may prescribe a stronger strength of steroids. Other agents your doctor may use to treat unrelenting itching are steroid pills or some classes of anti-depressants. Non-steroid creams, such as Elidel and Protopic, also help in the treatment of lichen simplex chronicus. To decrease the frequency of flares, women should moisturize the vulva daily and try to avoid stress and profuse sweating.

LICHEN SCLEROSUS

Vulvar lichen sclerosus (LS) is a chronic, progressive skin condition that mainly affects the genital area. LS is usually seen in females during phases of their life when estrogen is low, such as prior to puberty and in menopause. The cause of lichen sclerosus is unknown. However, a family history of the disease and disorders of the immune system are common in LS patients. Women with this condition complain of severe itching and pain of the vulva. Rarely, women with LS are without symptoms. On evaluation, white patches of skin are noted. With time, the skin becomes thin and crinkly, suggestive of an old cigarette paper appearance. The look is often called a "parchment-like" appearance. Women of color may have hyper (dark) or hypo (light) pigmented lesions. Because of the difference in appearance, women of color are often misdiagnosed. A delay in diagnosis and treatment can lead to long-term and sometimes permanent skin changes. As stated above, lichen sclerosus is a progressive disease. The changes in the vulvar architecture can lead to scarring and tightening of the vaginal opening, fissures or cracking along the labia and sometimes labial fusion (the labia sticking together). As you can imagine, women often develop painful sex. Many women are unable to have sex because of the pain. Painful urination is also common. The diagnosis of lichen sclerosis is made by biopsy. It is important to have a biopsy if LS is suspected and to keep at a minimum, yearly evaluation because LS can transition into vulvar cancer.

Overall, the risk of lichen sclerosus developing into cancer is less than five percent. The risk of cancer is decreased with early treatment and long-term management. The gold standard for treatment of this condition is a strong, topical steroid cream or ointment. Even if a woman's symptoms are mild, treatment is highly recommended. Early treatment decreases the risk of developing worsening lesions, including scarring or vulvar cancer. The initial treatment duration is six to twelve weeks. Afterwards, your doctor will taper the frequency of use to the lowest dose that keeps the lesion and symptoms from worsening. For example, some women may require weekly application of the steroid ointment to avoid the worsening of the disease, while others may need only monthly application. In women with an inadequate response to steroids, other treatment options, including a class of medications called calcineurin inhibitors and phototherapy, may be used. Women with severe adhesions and scarring may have disfigurement of the Private Face and limited function. With severe disease, surgery may be required to improve function and appearance.

Good hygiene practice helps to improve the quality of life in women living with LS. With thinning of the skin, extra steps should be taken to avoid further injury to the Private Face. Washing with a water or a mild soap is essential. Women with LS should avoid using a loofah.

Immediately after washing, a moisturizer should be applied to the vulva. Loose clothing will decrease friction. Panties with a narrow seat should be avoided. Normally, I'm telling you to wear cotton underwear. Women with LS should consider silk underwear. The silk will cause less friction to the skin compared to cotton. Unfortunately, silk is not as absorbable as cotton. If you choose to wear silk underwear when the weather outside is hot and humid, I recommend changing your undergarments more frequently. Women with LS should use lubrication with *every* sexual encounter. If you are not sexually active, consider using dilators with lubrication to help prevent the narrowing of the vaginal opening. If lichen sclerosus is negatively impacting your life, please consider finding a support group or meeting with a counselor. In the appendix, you will find a list of a few organizations that provide support to patients with lichen sclerosus. I strongly recommend a review of the support groups listed in the appendix of this book that can assist you in living with LS.

HIDRADENITIS SUPPURATIVA (HS)

Hidradenitis suppurativa is a benign, recurrent skin condition that can cause serious, long-term effects on a person's daily living. Many patients experience disruption to their emotional well-being. This disease process usually starts with small, painful bumps under the skin. These bumps can then become hard lumps, boils, or pus-filled abscesses and create raised sinus tracts or tunnels with chronic seepage under the skin. All these processes can damage the skin. HS is usually first seen after puberty. It mainly affects hairy areas of the skin that usually rub together, such as the armpits, groin area or even under the breasts.

The lumps of HS are found in areas where there are many hair follicles. Many hair follicles equal lots of oil and sweat glands. This combination is a perfect set-up for clogged pores. The lumps and sinus tract heal very slowly.

Due to the combination of oil and sweat glands being blocked, this can lead to pus formation. Again, the leakage of the pus can cause a nasty odor. Due to the possible connection of hormones, the severity of HS may lessen after menopause.

DIAGNOSIS:

    1) Having typical lesions or tracts

    2) Lesions noted in the typical locations

    3) Symptoms occurring for greater than six months

CAUSE

The true cause of HS is unknown. There are speculations about an association of this disease process and a malfunction of the immune system, hormones, and/or a mutation in an inherited gene. What we do know is that HS occurs secondary to blocked hair follicles and the apocrine sweat glands. If you have this condition, there is no need to feel ashamed. It is not caused by infection or poor hygiene. So, do not start vigorously scrubbing your external genitalia with the thoughts that you will cure this problem. Aggressive cleaning will only exacerbate the problem. In addition, HS is not contagious.

SYMPTOMS

1) **One or multiple red or flesh-colored bumps** – These bumps appear where there are many hair follicles.

2) **Bumps that look like blackheads having the "double barrel pattern"** – They can lead to pus formation. They appear as two dark spots beside each other. They give the appearance of the muzzle of a double-barrel shotgun.

3) **Painful bumps** – The initial presentation is one single, painful bump lasting for weeks. Subsequently, more bumps appear. These bumps often open to the skin surface, draining clear or yellow fluid.

4) **Sinus tracts** – These are raised tunnels under the skin

which connect the lesions. They initially start as abscess-like structures that transition into scarred tracts over time.

5) **Odor** – Many women experience an odor because of the overgrowth of bacteria.

RISK FACTORS

1) **Age** – HS is more likely to occur between the ages of 18 to 29. Research has shown that the earlier age of initial presentation increases your risk for widespread disease.

2) **Sex** – HS is more common in women. This could be secondary to the perceived hormonal connection.

3) **Race** – HS is more prevalent in people of color.

4) **Family History** – This supports the thought that there can be an inherited gene.

5) **Smoking** – Smoking increases your risk for almost everything! Again, quitting smoking is one of the single, most impactful lifestyle changes that people can make to markedly improve their overall health and quality of life.

6) **Obesity** – Since HS is most likely to be seen where skin rubs together, it is thought that obesity increases the frequency and friction of the skin connecting. Furthermore, obesity increases heat and sweat production, which can increase the risk of clogged pores.

7) **History of acne**

8) **Other medical conditions** – Crohn's disease, arthritis, inflammatory bowel disease, metabolic syndrome, or diabetes are all risk factors.

EXACERBATING FACTORS

Exacerbating factors are conditions that we can't control. These lifestyle choices can increase the frequency and severity of HS flares:

1) Obesity

2) Hormonal changes – including progesterone-only birth control

3) Heat and humidity

4) Metabolic syndrome

5) Stress

6) Smoking

7) Increased friction

COMPLICATIONS

1) **Infection** – The clogged pores contribute to the pooling of fluids produced by the sweat glands, which mixes with the bacteria attached to the hair follicles. The breakdown of the bumps also exposes the area to bacteria from the skin.

2) **Odor** – Let's not forget that the apocrine gland is one of the main sweat glands of the Private Face. Therefore, many people may develop an unpleasant odor.

3) **Skin changes** – Because of the inflammatory process and the connecting tunnels under the skin, many people develop significant scarring and hyperpigmentation. These skin changes can be long-term and permanent for some.

4) **Obstructed lymph drainage** – Our lymphatic system aids in the removal of toxins from the body. When this process is obstructed, the skin may show significant swelling.

5) **Restricted movement** – Movement in the affected area can be limited due to the scarring and pain.

6) **Social isolation** – HS in any area can lead to embarrassment. When HS involves the private face, not only can it be embarrassing, but it can markedly affect a woman's sexual experience. This type of emotional distress can affect every aspect of a woman's life, sometimes leading to sadness and even depression.

TREATMENT OPTIONS

There is no known cure for hidradenitis suppurativa. Treatment is aimed at reducing the recurrence and degree of damage with flares. The treatment of HS can be quite complex. Initiating treatment in the early phase can reduce long-term disease progression. Due to the aggressiveness of this condition, multiple treatment options are often initiated at the same time. Some patients with mild disease can treat the symptoms with lifestyle modifications and over-the-counter products. However, many women require prescription-strength medication and sometimes surgeries. The following is a list of common, but not all, treatment options:

1) **Mild, antibacterial wash** – This will be the only time that I tell you to use an antibacterial wash. This is due to the overabundance of bacteria present with this condition. The antibacterial wash will help reduce the odor caused by the bacteria.

2) **Warm baths or warm compresses**

3) **Steroid injections** – Kenalog is a steroid that can be injected directly into the lesion. The steroids decrease the pain related to the acute flare. The pain can be reduced within a day. Relief from inflammation may be noted within seven days.

4) **Antibiotics by mouth** – Antibiotics such as Clindamycin can be used to improve the microflora of the vulva. Such antibiotics also have anti-inflammatory properties.

5) **Anti-inflammatory pills**

6) **Anti-hormonals, such as Spironolactone**

7) **Retinoids** – One example is Accutane, which is usually reserved for moderate to severe cases.

8) **Biologics** – One example is Adalimumab (Humira). This is the only FDA-approved medication for the treatment of HS. Biologics work by modulating the immune system, thus controlling inflammation. This medication is reserved for the treatment of severe disease. For these patients, Adalimumab has been shown to be life-altering. Studies have shown up to 59 percent of patients achieving at least 50-percent reduction in total inflammatory lesions, with no new lesions or no new

sinus tract.[7]

9) **Surgery** – Surgery is the most effective treatment in HS that is refractory to other treatment options. The surgeries range from mild procedures of lancing and draining of the lesions to aggressive, extensive surgery, sometimes requiring skin grafting.

10) **Carbon dioxide laser therapy**

PREVENTATIVE MEASURES

There is no cure for HS. However, the following measures have been shown to improve the frequency of flares as well as the extent of disease:

1) **Proper counseling**

---

[7] Fotadou, C, Vakirlis E, Loannides D. Spotlight on adalimumab in the treatment of active moderate-to-severe hidradenitis suppurativa. Clin Cosmet Investig Dermatol. 2016; 9:367-372.

2) Reducing stimulation or friction to the hair follicles –
This can be accomplished in various ways. One of the most helpful benefits is for patients to STOP SHAVING the area. Women may also choose an alternative form of protection with menstruation instead of pads. No tweezing, picking or squeezing the area. All patients should wear loose clothing.

3) Weight reduction

4) Stop smoking

5) Changing contraception option – Progestin-only birth control options should be avoided.

6) Laser hair removal

7) HS support group – Please see the appendix at the back of the book.

8) Zinc supplementation

9) Vitamin C supplementation

10) Anti-inflammatories – Turmeric, honey, and apple cider vinegar are a few examples.

WHEN TO SEE THE DOCTOR

Every patient with suspected hidradenitis suppurativa should see a doctor immediately. The earlier you are given a diagnosis and initiate a treatment regimen, the better your chances are at avoiding long-term skin changes. Women with known or suspected HS should especially see a doctor for the following reasons:

1) Severe pain

2) No improvement in symptoms after a few weeks

3) A return of symptoms in a few short weeks after treatment

4) Lesions that appear in several locations

5) Frequent flares

BARTHOLIN'S CYST

As you learned earlier in the book, the Bartholin's glands are located slightly behind the opening of the vagina. They secrete fluid to lubricate the vagina. Sometimes, the opening of the gland can become blocked. The gland will then fill with fluid, and women develop a Bartholin's cyst. Women often complain of a painful bulging of the labia. Drainage from the cyst may be noted. An infected Bartholin's cyst is called an abscess. With infection, some women may develop fever. Bartholin's cyst may have an association with STDs. If you develop a Bartholin's cyst, I recommend an STD screen.

The treatment of Bartholin's cyst is usually simple. Warm sitz baths multiple times a day may resolve the cyst. Some cysts require surgical drainage. For recurrent cysts, a surgical procedure called marsupialization may be required. If an infection is present, antibiotics will also be given.

VULVAR CANCERS

Vulvar cancers most often affect the labia. They may also affect the clitoris or the Bartholin's glands. The most common type of vulvar cancers is squamous cell carcinomas.

These cancers make up about 90 percent of vulvar cancers. There are other types of vulvar cancers, too: some women may develop adenocarcinomas or melanomas. Metastatic disease may also present on the vulva.

Some women may experience a host of symptoms, while others may be asymptomatic. This adds to the importance of women actually *looking* at the Private Face. It is also imperative to keep up with yearly well-woman exams, even in the postmenopausal stage of life. The symptoms of vulvar cancer may include lumps or growths of the vulva, swollen lymph nodes in the groin or skin changes. Some women experience persistent itching, pain, soreness, or burning. Abnormal vaginal bleeding, ulcers of the vulva, pain with urination or wart-like growths may be signs of cancer. Please remember that changes to existing moles may also be a sign of vulvar cancer. Make sure that your healthcare provider is evaluating any moles at your annual exam. If you have been diagnosed with vulvar cancer, please go to the appendix of this book for a list of support groups

for women managing vulvar cancer.

CHAPTER 9

COMMON PROBLEMS OF THE VAGINA

The vagina is a very sensitive organ. Any irregularity in the vaginal area can be quite distressing. The smallest changes to the vagina have the potential to negatively impact a woman's quality of life. There are a host of common conditions that can affect the internal part of our Private Face. The different types of home remedies that women use to treat these various conditions are too numerous to count. Often, the measures used for symptom relief exacerbate the problem. The goal of this chapter is to give you a basic understanding of the common conditions that impact the vagina, as well as safe treatment options, prevention techniques, and the ability to know when a visit to the doctor is warranted.

VAGINAL DRYNESS

The majority of women experience vaginal dryness at some point in life. They may complain of vaginal itching or pain. Some women complain of a burning sensation or generalized soreness. The most common cause of vaginal dryness is the low estrogen levels found in postmenopausal women. The symptoms related to menopause will be discussed in Chapter 10. Here, I would like to discuss other causes of vaginal dryness. If you are experiencing vaginal dryness, pay attention to your medications. Some medications, such as antihistamines, can dry out the vagina. Often, using the wrong type of tampon can contribute to dryness. If you choose to use a super tampon when you are only experiencing mild vaginal bleeding, be prepared for your vagina to feel like a desert. Women with vaginal infections, such as yeast or even STDs, may have a dry vagina. Pay attention to your feminine hygiene products and detergents. A simple contact dermatitis can cause vaginal dryness. Last, but not least, prolonged or frequent vaginal intercourse can cause your vagina to feel like it's on fire. If you fall into this category, use a lubricant during sex. Consider taking a break from sex for at least a few days. You may also consider the use of coconut oil during your recovery phase. Coconut oil may provide moisture and promote healing of any small tears you may have received during your activities.

PAINFUL SEX AND THE VAGINA

My heart goes out to any woman who experiences painful sex. Intercourse is meant to be an enjoyable experience. If the cause for painful sex is not addressed, a woman can develop a complete aversion to sex. Problems with intercourse are a major cause of discord within relationships. In Chapter 7, we discussed the process of identifying the type of pain a woman develops with sex. Now, we will discuss the various types of painful sex that have a direct relationship with the vagina, their causes, and their treatment options.

SUPERFICIAL PAIN CAUSES

Inadequate vaginal lubrication – There are a host of reasons why a woman may experience decreased vaginal lubrication with sex. Some women simply need more foreplay. For others, the vaginal dryness is due to a lack of estrogen, which is commonly seen in menopause. Certain medications may also cause vaginal dryness. These include antihistamines, certain birth control pills, and high blood pressure medication. Some birth control pills can cause vaginal dryness. The blood pressure medications that affect lubrication are diuretics (or "water pills"), beta blockers, and alpha blockers.

Injury/irritation – Irritation to the vagina can occur from products such as soaps, bath bubbles, and bath salts. Some women have an allergy to various types of condoms or even semen. Some women experience pain after a birth injury or any surgery involving the vagina.

Infections – Infections such as yeast and bacterial vaginosis can contribute to painful sex. More importantly, sexually transmitted diseases (STDs) such as chlamydia, gonorrhea, or trichomoniasis can cause significant pain.

Congenital abnormalities – Some women are born with the absence of a fully formed vagina (vaginal agenesis) or a membrane blocking the opening of the vagina (imperforate hymen). These women will experience primary dyspareunia.

Vaginismus – Vaginismus is a condition that relates to the involuntary spasms of the vaginal muscles when anything is placed at the entry of the vagina. The spasms are caused by the fear of being hurt. This condition is sometimes seen in women with a history of sexual abuse.

DEEP PAIN CAUSES

Medical conditions – Conditions of the uterus itself can cause pain with deep penetration. These problems include uterine prolapse, retroverted uterus, uterine fibroids, and adenomyosis (overgrowth of the muscle of the uterus). Other conditions contributing to pain with deep penetration include endometriosis, pelvic inflammatory disease (PID), urinary tract infection, interstitial cystitis, irritable bowel syndrome, ovarian cysts, and pelvic floor dysfunction. These conditions are unrelated to the vagina, but important to mention. The vaginal factor that can cause pain with deep penetration is pelvic floor dysfunction. Most women refer to pelvic floor dysfunction as prolapse, or pelvic organ prolapse.

Previous surgeries – Surgeries can cause scar tissue to develop. The scar tissue contributes to deep penetration pain. After a total hysterectomy, some women may have a shortened vagina. Due to the decrease in the vaginal length, women may develop secondary dyspareunia.

Partner – Penile size is a common cause of deep dyspareunia. Partners with delayed orgasms may also contribute to a woman's pain.

Radiation/chemotherapy – These agents can cause significant scarring of the pelvis, which leads to pain with intercourse.

TREATMENT OPTIONS

As stated in Chapter 7, treatment of painful sex depends on the cause of the pain. Inadequate lubrication can be treated by being more mindful of foreplay. Your healthcare provider may consider changing your birth control method or blood pressure medication. Local and systemic estrogen therapy can be used to build up the lining of the vagina, which will improve vaginal lubrication. Lidocaine gel or ointment can be used at the vestibule.

Injuries of the vagina can cause pain with intercourse for an extended period of time. It is important to delay sex until injuries after childbirth and surgery are healed, because even if you're not feeling pain while resting, the vaginal mucosa may not be completely recovered. Pelvic rest – or more bluntly, the avoidance of anything in the vagina – is the primary treatment for painful sex caused by vaginal deliveries or surgery.

If you are experiencing vaginal irritation with condom use, that is not an excuse for unprotected sex in high-risk situations. If you suspect an allergy to condoms, try a latex-free option. There are condoms made of various products, including sheep's skin. The same process holds true for vaginal lubrications. Try different types if you think you are having a reaction to your current lubricant.

Any possibility of infection should be immediately evaluated and treated with antibiotics. Pelvic rest is necessary until treatment for yeast or bacterial vaginosis is completed. If you are diagnosed with a sexually transmitted disease (STD), pelvic rest should occur for two weeks. It is imperative that your partner is treated and that there is no intercourse until both partners have reached two weeks since treatment. The last thing you want to do is re-introduce infection.

Birth defects may not be diagnosed until after the first sexual experience. Those with vaginal agenesis (no fully formed vagina) may be treated with vaginal dilators, but most require surgery. The imperforate hymen (membrane over the vaginal opening) is treated with a simple, outpatient procedure. Surgery or dilators may not always resolve dyspareunia. For these women, emotional support and counseling are imperative.

The involuntary muscle contractions called vaginismus may require more than one treatment modality to gain pain-free sex. The treatment goal for vaginismus is to relax the muscles of the pelvic floor. Pelvic floor exercises are very effective. Dilators and manual touch can be used to desensitize the vagina. Due to fear and likely previous sexual abuse, psycho-social counseling is the cornerstone to treatment of vaginismus. The appendix in the back of this book provides a list of support groups for women living with vaginismus.

Surgery may be required to treat conditions such as uterine fibroids, adenomyosis, endometriosis, interstitial cystitis, ovarian cysts, and pelvic adhesions (scar tissue). A shortened vagina after hysterectomy cannot be reversed. However, some women may have improvement in pain with estrogen cream and serial dilator use. If the pain with intercourse is related to the size of your partner, consider trying different positions with sex. If your partner suffers with delayed ejaculation, vaginal lubrication should be helpful.

If there is an emotional component to painful sex, behavioral modifications are helpful. Women can employ a sex therapist to help with their experience. Women with mental disease or a history of abuse should consider a counselor, psychologist, and/or a psychiatrist. Emotional support can be used along with other treatment modalities.

WHEN TO SEE A DOCTOR:

If the pain with intercourse is persistent, it is important to be seen by your doctor. Women also need to be seen if they are experiencing abnormal bleeding with the pain. If there is new onset of vaginal discharge, a pelvic exam is warranted. STD screening must occur if there is a possibility of infection. If there are any skin lesions or sores inside of the vagina, do not delay an appointment with your doctor.

THE SMELL DOWN THERE AND THE VAGINA

What about the smell down there? Is it common to have an odor? Well, a slight odor is very normal. Every woman has a unique smell. You should be evaluated if your smell changes abruptly or if there is a fishy, foul-smelling odor. There are many factors that can affect the smell down there. We will cover the common issues that can turn your nose up and your smile upside down.

FACTORS THAT INFLUENCE SMELL

Poor hygiene – The number one factor to smell is hygiene. We all know that the vagina is a self-cleaning organ. However, the odor that women sometimes experience does not come from the vagina. The odor usually comes from the natural vaginal discharge that is left in the folds and crevices of the outside portion of the Private Face. Therefore, it is important for this area to be washed. Some may say to wash only with water, and that's perfectly okay. If you choose to use soap, select a mild soap. This is where the pH comes into play. The pH of the wash needs to be consistent with the pH of the vagina and vulva. Some products may display slogans such as "Ph balanced for women". Others may not mention the Ph. It is completely up to the manufacturer if they chose to mention anything about the Ph of their product. If you're curious, consider purchasing some Ph sticks. You can find them online and sometimes at your local pet store. After washing, the area must be dry. Again, incomplete drying leads to a warm, moist environment. Such an environment is the perfect setup for a yeast infection.

Hydration – When we are not well hydrated, the smell of our vaginal discharge will be more concentrated. It's amazing what eight glasses of water per day can do.

Diet – Certain foods can also impact the smell down there. Strong spices such as curry can seep from the pores of the body, including the vagina. We will touch more on diet in Chapter 11.

Infection – Infections such as bacterial vaginosis and trichomoniasis can lead to a foul, fishy odor. It is the anaerobic bacteria of these infections that causes the smell. Anaerobic bacteria are bugs that can survive without oxygen.

Retained tampons - Retained tampons can become a source of infection. As bacteria grows on the tampon inside the vagina, a horrible odor can ensue. Sometimes, the odor is only noticed with sex. If you think you may have retained a tampon, it is important to remove it immediately. First, wash your hands. Then, try squatting, relax the body, and feel for the string with one finger. If you are unable to remove the tampon, ask your partner, or make an appointment with your medical provider. If you develop fever, chills, nausea, vomiting, a rash on the soles of your feet or the palms of your hands, headaches, muscle aches, confusion, or seizures, seek medical attention immediately.

VAGINAL DISCHARGE

One of the most common areas of concern for women is vaginal discharge. As discussed in Chapter 4, some vaginal discharge is normal. The challenge for most women is distinguishing the normal from the abnormal. Normal discharge can appear white or clear. The consistency can be thin like milk or thicker like mucus. Discharge is normally thin and sometimes sticky early in your menstrual cycle. It may become more pronounced and mucus-like during ovulation. Normal discharge may be odorless or slightly scented. Every woman has a unique smell. It is important to become acquainted with your normal smell. Any changes to the normal characteristics of your vaginal discharge should be deemed as abnormal. If the color changes to yellow, green, gray, or brown, consider the discharge to be abnormal.

If the consistency changes to thick and curdy or if there is a large amount of discharge, an evaluation is warranted. Unrelated to sex, there should not be a large amount of discharge. Vaginal discharge should never be fishy or foul smelling.

CAUSES OF ABNORMAL DISCHARGE

I like to refer to the female genitalia as a garden. The external genitalia has its own garden, and then there is the garden of the vagina. The vaginal garden is the vaginal microbiome. The vaginal microbiome or flora consists of healthy microorganisms or bugs that help to keep the vagina healthy. So, in your vaginal garden, you have beautiful flowers that promote community wellness. There may be a few weeds or bad bugs that we can live with. Abnormal discharge develops when the weeds start to overgrow in your garden. Now, let's talk about some of the weeds that cause abnormal discharge.

VAGINAL CANDIDIASIS

Vaginal candidiasis is most commonly referred to as a yeast infection. Yeast is a fungus that is commonly found in your vaginal garden in small amounts. The yeast becomes an infection when it begins to overgrow or when it penetrates deeper vaginal layers. There are multiple types of fungus that can cause a yeast infection. The most common fungus found with vaginal yeast infections is Candida albicans.

Women with vaginal candidiasis usually experience vaginal irritation, itching and burning. They may have redness and swelling of the vagina. The discharge associated with vaginal yeast infections is thick, white and odor-free. Yeast infections may have the classic cottage cheese appearance, or may appear watery.

RISK FACTORS:

A host of conditions may increase your risk for yeast infections. Certain classes of antibiotics, such as penicillins, tetracyclines, or quinolones, may increase your risk for infection. Women who are pregnant or suffer from conditions such as uncontrolled diabetes mellitus or an impaired immune system may be more prone from vaginal candidiasis. Medications such as steroids, birth control pills or hormonal therapy with increased estrogen levels can increase your risk for yeast infections. The first experience of vaginal intercourse is also a risk factor for vaginal candidiasis.

TREATMENT OPTIONS:

It is perfectly okay to use OTC antifungals for yeast infections. These treatment options usually consist of a single dose, or up to a seven-day course, of treatment. Prescriptions are also given for yeast infections. Treatment may consist of creams, ointments, pills, or suppositories. Complicated cases of yeast may be treated with longer regimens of antifungals or with boric acid suppositories.

Boric acid comes from the natural compound called boron. It is an antifungal and mild antiseptic. It helps to rid the disease-causing organism (in this case, yeast). In reference to your vaginal garden, you can consider boric acid as a weed killer that is bought at your local gardening store. Boric acid does not require a prescription. It is used as a vaginal suppository. Boric acid should **never** be ingested. Swallowing boric acid can lead to death. Even if a medication does not require a prescription, I recommend consulting with your healthcare provider prior to placing anything in the vagina.

PREVENTION:

Many yeast infections are preventable. Healthy habits such as wearing cotton-seat underwear, loose clothing and avoiding prolonged exposure to wet clothes (i.e. bathing suits) can help to prevent yeast infections. Women should avoid hot baths, hot tubs, and douching. Women should also avoid unnecessary use of antibiotics. A more robust discussion of healthy habits for vaginal health are found in Chapter 12.

WHEN TO SEE A DOCTOR:

If this is your first experience with a possible yeast infection, a visit with your doctor is recommended. If your symptoms are unrelieved with over-the-counter medications or if you are unsure of your diagnosis, a pelvic exam is needed. All women with complicated yeast should be evaluated by their healthcare provider. Complicated yeast consists of extensive redness, swelling, or itching that has led to tears, cracks, or sores. Recurrent yeast infections are considered complicated. Women with health conditions such as pregnancy, uncontrolled diabetes, or a weak immune system, as with HIV, should be seen by a doctor.

BACTERIAL VAGINOSIS

Another common cause of abnormal vaginal discharge is bacterial vaginosis, most commonly known as BV. The fancy name for BV is Gardnerella vaginalis. BV is yet another weed in your vaginal garden. This condition occurs when there is loss of vaginal lactobacilli (good bugs) and an overgrowth of Gardnerella (bad bugs). In reference to your vaginal garden, consider lactobacilli as your vagina's natural weed killer. Lactobacilli produces hydrogen peroxide, which boosts the body's immune system and its ability to fight bad bugs and other foreign organisms.

Women with bacterial vaginosis may complain of vaginal pain, itching or burning. The discharge with BV is usually thin, white, or gray. The most common complaint from women with bacterial vaginosis is a fishy vaginal odor. The odor is most pronounced after sex.

RISK FACTORS:

There are many factors that can increase your risk for bacterial vaginosis. The number one risk for bacterial vaginosis is a lack of hydrogen peroxide producing lactobacilli. Vaginal intercourse increases your risk for BV. The risk is greater with anal sex before vaginal intercourse, sex with an uncircumcised male partner, and the use of vaginal lubricants. Keep in mind that alkaline semen can raise the vaginal pH and increase your risk for BV. Semen has a natural pH between 7.1-8. Other risk factors are vitamin D deficiency, smoking, and race (Black women are more at risk). We will discuss the risk of BV in Black women separately.

TREATMENT OPTIONS:

Mild cases of bacterial vaginosis may resolve without treatment. In general, BV is treated with antibiotics. The medication may be given as pills or as vaginal inserts or suppositories. Male partners of women with bacterial vaginosis do not require treatment. However, BV can be transferred between female partners. The treatment of bacterial vaginosis decreases the risk of sexually transmitted diseases. Recurrent BV can be treated with adding boric acid suppositories as a supplement to antibiotic therapy.

COMPLICATIONS OF BV:

Bacterial vaginosis increases the risk of sexually transmitted diseases by weakening the barrier membrane of the vagina. BV can cause preterm deliveries and increased risk for post-surgical complications. Rarely, bacterial vaginosis can lead to pelvic inflammatory disease (PID). PID occurs when an infection in the vagina ascends into other pelvic organs, such as the uterus, tubes, ovaries, and the bowels. Pelvic inflammatory disease can cause severe pain. Some women may develop abscesses in their tubes and ovaries, or even infection in the blood stream. PID is a known

171

cause of infertility.

PREVENTION TECHNIQUES:

Prevention of bacterial vaginosis starts with good Private Face hygiene. I cannot stress enough about cotton-seat underwear and the avoidance of douching. You will learn all about good hygiene habits in Chapter 12. Due to the association of bacterial vaginosis and STDs, safe sex is essential. Daily probiotic supplements can help treat and prevent bacterial vaginosis. Yogurt also contains natural probiotics. I recommend one serving of yogurt per day if you are prone to developing bacterial vaginosis. In Chapter 11 we will have a great discussion about how your diet affects the health of your vagina. Another healthy preventative measure is adding hydrogen peroxide to your bath water or using it as a sitz bath. Garlic is known to have antibacterial properties. Garlic supplementation may be beneficial in preventing BV. There is one study that shows that vaginal creams with garlic improve bacterial vaginosis.[8] Clearly, I am all about healthy vaginas. I don't know about you, but the thought of my vagina smelling like garlic really doesn't work for me. Lastly, every woman with the diagnosis of bacterial vaginosis should check their vitamin D level.

BLACK WOMEN AND BV:

Black women are three times as likely as white women to have bacterial vaginosis.[9] Black women are also more prone to develop recurrent infections. With the added factors of historical wrongs and negative stereotypes, many Black women suffering with bacterial vaginosis carry

---

[8] Khalifa Soltani M. More study of garlic extract. Pharmacist thesis...: Esfahan University of Medical Sciences; 1992.

[9] Allsworth JE, Peipert JF. Prevalence of bacterial vaginosis: 2001-2004. National Health and Nutrition Examination Survery data. Obstet Gynecol. 2007; 109:114-20.

additional shame. Often, their only information in reference to BV is the association with poor hygiene practices, lower socioeconomic status, sexual frequency, and sexually transmitted diseases. The additional shame contributes to some women aggressively cleaning the Private Face, which in turn causes more harm. For many Black women, there is a negative impact on their sexual experiences. They stop having sex because of the embarrassment of the odor or the fear of recurrent infections. Well, I'm here to tell you that there is more to BV in Black women, and there are treatment options.

The microbiome, or vaginal garden, in Black women is slightly different than the garden of white women. First, the vaginal pH of Black women is slightly higher than white women's. The increased pH alone increases the risk for bacterial vaginosis. We previously talked about lactobacilli being the vagina's natural weed killer. When it comes to lactobacilli, Black women have been given the one-two punch. First, black women are more likely to have a vaginal pH greater than 4.5 and no lactobacilli. Secondly, the predominant type of lactobacilli seen in Black women is different from that seen in white women. The predominant lactobacilli in white women are Lactobacillus crispatus, which is associated with a lower pH. We already know that a lower pH promotes a healthy vagina. Black women are dominated with Lactobacillus iners, which often has a higher pH.[10] With these negative punches in mind, more research needs to be done specifically about Black women and BV at the molecular level. In other areas, while notable research has been completed, the knowledge obtained from these studies has unfortunately not reached the masses. One significant study was done at the University of Pittsburgh and reported

---

[10] Hummelen R, Fernandes AD, Macklaim JM, Dickson RJ, Changalucha J, Gloor GB, Reid G: Deep sequencing of the vaginal microbiota of women with HIV: PLoS ONE. 2010; 8:e 12078.

in 2009. The study found that Black women are nearly three times more likely as white women to have a vitamin D deficiency, which is linked to an increased risk of bacterial vaginosis.[11] Let me repeat this statement plainly. Vitamin D deficiency increases the risk for bacterial vaginosis! Who is at increased risk for vitamin D deficiency? Black women! Dark skin pigmentation inhibits the sun's ability to make vitamin D3. Another significant conclusion from this study was that white women who had low levels of vitamin D were as likely to have bacterial vaginosis as Black women.

How many women with recurrent bacterial vaginosis have been made aware of this association? How many of you have received the recommendation to check your vitamin D

---

[11] Bodnar LM, Krohn MA, Simhan HN. Maternal Vitamin D Deficiency Is Associated with Bacterial Vaginosis in the First Trimester of Pregnancy. The Journal of Nutrition, volume 139, Issue 6, June 2009, pages 1157-1161.

level by the healthcare provider managing your vitamin D? My goal with this book is to give you enough information to advocate for yourself. Never forget that education is your most powerful weapon.

CHAPTER 10

MEDICAL PROBLEMS OF THE VAGINA

Medical problems of the vagina are often overlooked and ignored. A large reason for many undiagnosed or late discoveries of medical conditions involving the vagina are because women are uncomfortable with embracing the Private Face. The second reason for delay in management is the lack of education. Early diagnosis and treatment are the key to preventing long-term complications. Here we will discuss the most common medical problems of the vagina.

STDs AND THE VAGINA

Sexually transmitted diseases (STDs) are the most common vaginal condition in reproductive-aged women. STDs may include trichomoniasis, chlamydia, gonorrhea, and HIV infection. Herpes and syphilis were covered in Chapter 8. Some women may complain of vaginal irritation, vaginal pain, soreness, vaginal discharge, or pelvic pain. Other women may be without symptoms. This adds to the need for annual STD screenings until you are one year past marriage, and especially if you are participating in high-risk behavior. I consider high-risk behavior as unprotected sex with a new partner without recent, documented testing; receiving anal sex; having more than one sexual partner; being sexually involved with an unfaithful partner (especially if suspected of performing anal sex); and being sexually involved with a partner who was recently incarcerated. It is important to complete all medication given for infection and to inform your partner(s). Please refrain from sex until both parties have been treated for two weeks. Untreated STDs can lead to infertility or pelvic inflammatory disease, including severe infection. Human immunodeficiency virus (HIV) can cause a host of medical conditions, secondary infections, and cancers secondary to a poor immune system.

MENOPAUSE

Menopause occurs when a woman has gone without menses or bleeding for one year. It is caused by the reduction in estrogen that occurs as a woman grows older. There is also surgical menopause. This type of menopause is secondary to the surgical removal of the ovaries. Without the ovaries, women are unable to produce estrogen. The terms "menopause" and "postmenopausal" essentially have the same meaning. These terms will be used interchangeably. The changes of the Private Face over time were discussed in Chapter 6. Here, we will discuss these changes in more detail, as well as potential treatment options.

During menopause, women lose muscle tone and are at risk of the weakening of the pelvic floor. Such pelvic relaxation can lead to prolapse or dropping of the bladder, uterus and/or bowels. Women who have experienced multiple vaginal deliveries or delivery of large infants are more prone to this condition. Some women experience leaking urine with coughing or sneezing, feeling pressure in the vagina or difficulty with bowel movements. In severe cases, women can see and feel a protrusion from the vagina. Prolapse is usually managed with surgery. Women who are poor candidates for surgery may be offered placement of a pessary into the vagina.

The decreased production of estrogen and even testosterone (although to a lesser extent) during menopause can cause a host of irritating, stress-provoking, and sometimes debilitating symptoms. This condition is known as genitourinary syndrome of menopause (GMS). Women develop symptoms such as vulvar dryness and burning, vaginal dryness, and pain with intercourse. GSM may also cause urinary problems, including painful urination, urinary urgency, and urinary tract infections. It has been reported that genitourinary syndrome can be seen in up to 50 percent of postmenopausal women.[12] The percent of women affected may be underreported. Too many women feel ashamed or embarrassed to report such concerns to their healthcare provider. Some women feel that reporting any symptoms in reference to the Private Face is counter-productive because they assume that there are no treatment options. Unfortunately, too many women are suffering in silence. The good news is that there are multiple treatment options. Even though genitourinary syndrome is mainly due to low estrogen, there are both hormonal and non-hormonal treatment options.

---

[12] Crean-Tate K, Faubion SS, Pederson H, Vencill J, Batur P: Management of genitourinary syndrome of menopause in female cancer patients: a focus on vaginal hormonal therapy. American Journal of Obstetrics and Gynecology, volume 222, issue 2, February 2020, pages P103-113.

NON-HORMONAL TREATMENT OPTIONS

Vaginal moisturizers – Vaginal moisturizers should be used regularly for maintenance therapy. They help to hydrate the lining of the vagina and lower the pH. Some women experience vaginal irritation even without having sex. These moisturizers can be used with and without sex.

Vaginal lubricants – Lubricants provide a barrier between the vagina and penis to reduce friction. They are used to relieve pain with intercourse.

Topical anesthetics – Women with moderate to severe painful intercourse can use local anesthetics, such as Lidocaine, at the vaginal opening. The medication needs to be applied at least three minutes prior to penetration.

Pelvic floor physical therapy – Some physical therapists specialize in pelvic floor dysfunction. Through pelvic floor biofeedback, exercises to strengthen and relax the pelvic floor, and manual manipulations, women can see an improvement in pain with intercourse and orgasm.

Vaginal laser and radiofrequency rejuvenation – Both laser and radiofrequency heat up the vaginal tissues, resulting in increased collagen formation. They result in significant improvement in vaginal pain, dryness, and pain with intercourse.

O Shot/G Shot – The O shot is also called the orgasm shot. It is created by taking platelet rich plasma from your own blood. The plasma is injected into the clitoris. This stimulates blood flow and cell growth, which in turn improves a woman's orgasm. The G shot is an injection of hyaluronic acid base filler. It is injected into the Grafenberg spot, affectionately known as the G spot. Think of the G spot as the Hot Spot or Happy Spot. It is an erogenous zone on the roof of the vagina, right below the urethra. This injection is for women who have lost their ability to orgasm, or for those who desire to improve the quantity or quality of the experience.

HORMONAL TREATMENT OPTIONS

Vaginal estrogen therapy – Low-dose vaginal estrogen therapy has been shown to improve vaginal thickness, lubrication, and the associated pain with intercourse. Estrogen helps to lower the vaginal pH and decrease the occurrence of urinary tract infections. Women with heart disease or a history of blood clots can safely use low-dose estrogen therapy because of its low rate of systemic absorption.

Vaginal DHEA (Prasterone) – DHEA improves vaginal secretions, thickness, and collagen formation. In general, Prasterone can improve vaginal health and sexual function via desire, arousal, lubrication, and orgasm.

Vaginal testosterone – Vaginal testosterone has been found to improve vaginal assessment scores, lower the vaginal pH, and improve the vaginal flora. Improving the vaginal flora helps to decrease the occurrence of infections. Testosterone also improves vaginal dryness and pain with intercourse.

Systemic estrogen therapy – Systemic estrogen therapy is often simply called "hormone replacement therapy," or HRT. Women who no longer have a uterus can use estrogen alone. Women with a uterus must use progesterone in addition to estrogen to protect the lining of the uterus from cancer. Systemic estrogen therapy is not as effective as local estrogen therapy in the treatment of genitourinary syndrome of menopause (GSM). However, women who have additional menopausal symptoms, such as hot flashes, may benefit from traditional hormone replacement therapy.

Please remember that HRT is contraindicated in women with a history of heart disease, stroke, uncontrolled high blood pressure, uncontrolled diabetes, blood clots, or hormone-related cancers. Discuss with your provider all of the contraindications and risks of this medication prior to use.

Selective estrogen receptor modulators (SERM)

Ospemifene (or Osphena) is a medication that manipulates estrogen receptors in the body. It provides the same effect on the vagina as estrogen. Osphena is FDA-approved for the treatment of moderate to severe vaginal dryness and painful intercourse due to menopause. Its use is contraindicated in women with a history of heart disease, stroke, or blood clots. Discuss with your provider all of the contraindications and risks of this medication prior to use.

LICHEN PLANUS

Lichen planus is an inflammatory skin condition that can affect both the vulva and vagina. It affects 0.5-2 percent of the population. Lichen planus is mainly seen in women in their fifties and sixties. Women usually experience vulvar pain, vaginal pain, burning, itching, soreness, and painful sex. Different from the other vulvar skin condition discussed in Chapter 8, women with lichen planus may have an irritating vaginal discharge and bleeding after sex. A small subset of women may not have symptoms.

Lichen planus usually appears as a well-defined, bright red patch or ulcer. These areas on the skin can cause structural changes to the genitalia, including loss of the labia minora and narrowing of the vaginal opening. The diagnosis is made by biopsy. This condition can present in other areas of the body, including the mouth, scalp, nails, and anus. The true cause of lichen planus is unknown. It is thought to be caused by a disruption in the immune system. If you are diagnosed with this condition, your doctor will look for other autoimmune disorders.

There is no cure for vulvar lichen planus. However, the condition can be managed with early diagnosis, conscientious hygiene practices, use of dilators, topical anesthetics, topical estrogen, chronic use of steroid therapy, and sometimes surgery. Due to the symptoms associated with lichen planus and its permanent existence once diagnosed, it is important for women to have a strong support system.

CANCER OF THE VAGINA

Primary vaginal cancer is rare. Cancers that originate from other areas are more often seen in women. Some women may not have symptoms early in the disease. Women with vaginal cancer may develop postmenopausal bleeding or bleeding after sex. Some women may experience a watery discharge. Women with advanced disease may notice a mass in the vagina, urinary symptoms, pelvic pain, and even constipation. If you are experiencing any of the symptoms associated with vaginal cancer, please schedule an appointment with your healthcare provider. Any woman with a history of dysplasia of the vagina (vaginal intraepithelial neoplasia, or VAIN) or exposure to diethylstilbestrol (DES) while in her mother's womb is at increased risk for vaginal cancer. Women who are smokers and/or HIV positive are at risk for developing vaginal cancer. To prevent this disease and to avoid a delay in diagnosis, please continue to obtain your annual exams, even if you are not due for a pap smear. We use a speculum to collect a pap smear and also to examine the lining of the vagina. Your healthcare provider will likely look at your vagina every year. It allows us the opportunity to identify any abnormal bumps, sores or lesions that cannot be seen by looking in the mirror.

PHASE 3: PAMPER THE PRIVATE FACE

CHAPTER 11

THE IMPACT OF DIET ON THE PRIVATE FACE

We as women have often been taught that the health of our Private Face is controlled by either placing products on the vulva or inside of the vagina. Women want to know if it is possible to control the smell and taste of the vagina. They want to know the possible measures to decrease ingrown hairs, improve their vaginal dryness or guarantee overall sexual experience. However, rarely is there a discussion about how one's diet affects the Private Face. A healthy diet has the greatest impact on the Private Face, as well as a woman's overall health. Diet modifications can have both a negative and positive impact on the Private Face.

NEGATIVE DIETARY MEASURES

The following are negative dietary measures:

Dehydration

Dehydration can lead to overall dryness of the vulva and vagina. It can also make any vaginal odor more pronounced. As I have said multiple times in this book, women should drink at least eight glasses of water per day.

Alcohol

Alcohol consumption is okay if done with moderation. Increased alcohol consumption leads to increased water loss through urination, which leads to dehydration.

Too Much Sugar

Sugary foods and drinks will increase your blood glucose levels. This will increase your risk for yeast infections. Too many refined carbohydrates can also cause this problem.

Examples of refined carbohydrates are white flour, white bread, and breakfast cereals.

High Fat Foods

High fat foods, such as fried foods and excessive consumption of cheese, can disrupt your vaginal pH. Fatty foods can also increase your risk for bacterial vaginosis.

Stinky Veggies

Certain vegetables are good for your health, but over-consumption can lead to an unpleasant vaginal smell. If you are anticipating a special night, try to avoid asparagus, broccoli, onions, and garlic for lunch and dinner. Strong-smelling spices, such as curry, can also cause this problem.

POSITIVE DIETARY MEASURES

While there are negative dietary measures, there are also positive ones. They include:

Water

Water is essential for the maintenance of your beauty below the waist.

Cranberries

Cranberries are a great source of antioxidants, which fight age-related damage to tissues. They are also bactericidal. By killing bugs in the bladder, they help prevent urinary tract infections (UTIs).

Probiotics

Probiotics promote both digestive and vaginal health. They help control the pH balance of the vagina by promoting the growth of "good" bugs. Probiotics are also a great source of calcium, which helps to decrease PMS symptoms.

Sweet Potatoes

Sweat potatoes are an excellent source of beta-carotenes and Vitamin A. They help to brighten the skin of the vagina, prevent ingrown hairs, strengthen the uterine walls, and improve fertility.

Phytoestrogens

Phytoestrogens are natural compounds that mimic estrogens. A common phytoestrogen is soy. Examples of foods high in soy are edamame, tempeh, and tofu. The isoflavones in soy improve the health of skin and blood vessels. The improvement in blood flow decreases vaginal dryness.

Fruits

Many fruits have a positive impact on the Private Face. Here is a small example of how various fruits can impact the Private Face: apples contain a phytoestrogen that improves sexual function. Avocado is also a fruit. It contains healthy fats: Vitamin B6 and potassium. Avocados help to increase lubrication and strengthen the vaginal walls. Pineapples have a lot of Vitamin C, antioxidants, and anti-inflammatory properties. Mangoes promote growth and repair. Papayas are full of Vitamin A, which promotes healthy hair and skin. They also contain Vitamin C, antioxidants, fiber, folate, and anti-inflammatory properties.

Dark, leafy greens

Dark leafy greens such as kale, collards, and spinach improve the circulation of blood. The improved circulation at the vaginal level results better lubrication and improved stimulation. These greens are also full of Vitamin E, magnesium, and calcium. Vitamin E is a great antioxidant. It protects cells from damage and slows the aging process. Calcium is great for your muscles and nerves, including the pelvic floor muscles. Magnesium is an essential mineral for muscle movement and the nervous system. It also has anti-inflammatory proprieties. Magnesium can improve exercise performance, even in the bedroom.

THE PRIVATE FACE SMOOTHIE

I created the Private Face Smoothie to give women a simple and tasteful option to promote optimal beauty below the waistline. It is recommended to drink the smoothie three times per week. The smoothie is an excellent meal replacement, especially in the mornings. The coconut water and oil are used because they are excellent for hydration and vaginal lubrication. The Vitamin A in the coconut also helps with preventing ingrown hair. Manuka honey has been found to promote wound healing. It also contains antibacterial, antioxidant and anti-inflammatory properties.

Ingredients:

½ cup of coconut water

1 handful of stemless spinach

2 teaspoons of manuka honey

1 tablespoon of coconut oil

½ cup of 100% cranberry juice

4 oz of Activia

½ cup of almond milk (vanilla flavor preferred)

1 kiwi

1 cup of mango, pineapple, or papaya

Directions:

Blend the coconut water and spinach until a smooth consistency is achieved. Add the Manuka honey, the coconut oil and blend. Add the cranberry juice, Activia and almond milk and blend. Add fruit and blend.

CHAPTER 12

HEALTHY HABITS FOR THE PRIVATE FACE

As you read throughout this book, you find that certain lifestyle habits increase your risk for almost every condition that affects the Private Face. Let's dig deeper into proper hygiene of the Private Face.

CLOTHING SELECTION

How many times have the preventative measures included wearing loose clothes? I can't say it enough. If it's too tight, it's not right for the Private Face. Our special area needs to be able to breathe. Snug clothes will not only increase heat and sweat. They contribute to the blockage of your pores or hair follicles. We already know what happens when those follicles are blocked.

Many feel that the G-string is cute. But ask yourself: is that cute, little, tiny piece of fabric worth causing trauma to your precious skin, or creating a home for bacteria to grow? I'm assuming the answer is no. Consider going without underwear at night. This is the perfect time to allow the area to breathe.

RESTROOM HABITS

Another recurring theme of vulvar vaginal health is proper hygiene. Restroom habits are extremely important. This is the moment throughout the day when the Private Face is potentially exposed to unhealthy bacteria. Those bad bugs are right next door. It is important that after urinating, we are wiping front to back. Send the bad bugs away from the Private Face! With ensuring cleanliness, don't wipe too hard. It doesn't take much to be clean. Aggressive wiping will cause more harm than good. With defecation, the same principle applies. Granted, sometimes it's a little harder to remove all the remnants. Some people use wipes to fix this. Wipes are okay if used properly, but first, look at the ingredients. Make sure that there are no ingredients that could potentially be harmful to the Private Face. Try to stay away from wipes with an added fragrance unless it is a high quality, natural fragrance. You can learn more about fragrances in Chapter 11's Product Selection Guide. Still, make sure you are not too aggressive. After using the wipes, pat the area dry with toilet paper.

Another recurring theme is to keep the Private Face dry, so an alternative to using wet wipes is using a spray bottle filled with water. Even with the spray bottle, allow the area to either air dry, or blot with toilet paper.

WASHING AND POST-WASHING TECHNIQUES

Recommendations for washing the Private Face have become a highly debated topic. For the most part, all parties agree that the vagina is a self-cleaning organ. There is no need to place anything into the vagina to clean it. The debate comes into play when discussing the proper way to clean the external genitalia. Some feel that only water should be used. They also feel that the area should only be cleaned with hands. Others feel that it is okay to use mild soaps.

If a woman wants to use only water, I have no objections. If she wants to use her hands, that's okay with me, too. However, I don't feel that there is anything wrong with using a mild soap or a soft washcloth. The key is being gentle and getting into those crevices. The crevices are where the vaginal discharge likes to accumulate. If that material is lodged within all your nooks and crannies, then over time, bacteria will grow and become stinky. In my opinion, it could be a little difficult removing that residue with only your hand and water. In summary, the following items are needed to properly wash the Private Face:

WASHING AGENTS

Water – Water is okay to use if you are not removing your pubic hairs or you do not have any vulvar skin condition such as pseudo-folliculitis barbae or hidradenitis suppurativa.

Mild soap – It is okay for anyone to use a mild soap.

WASHING INSTRUMENTS

Your hand – It is okay to wash with only your hands if you are not removing your pubic hairs. If you choose to use your hands, please be mindful of the sharpness of your fingernails.

Washcloth – Make sure to thoroughly rinse and hang your washcloth after each use. The washcloth should be changed at least every three days.

Shower loofah – In general, shower loofahs are okay to use. I caution their use in the non-hairy areas of the labia minora. They may cause irritation. It is important to thoroughly rinse and hang the loofah after each use for complete drying. A sponge loofah should be replaced every month. A mesh loofah can be changed every two months.

Shower glove – The shower glove is the gold standard for cleaning the Private Face. The glove should have different textures on each side. The rougher side is for exfoliation. This side should only have a small degree of roughness. It is used for exfoliating the mons pubis and labia majora. The smoother side should be used for the labia minora. Some women will also use the smooth side on the labia majora. Make sure to rinse the shower glove thoroughly after each use. Hang the glove outside of the shower to decrease the exposure to additional moisture. Let's not forget that bacteria love to grow in warm, most areas. The shower glove should be washed or replaced every month.

POST-WASHING TECHNIQUES

Going back to the recurring themes, keeping the Private Face dry promotes good vulvar and vaginal health. After bathing, make sure that the Private Face is blotted dry. Once again, *no aggressive rubbing*! Make sure that you are hanging your bath towel after use. For my teenage patients, this has proven to be quite difficult. Damp towels left on the floor or on the counter are bad news for the Private Face. If you are overweight, extra attention needs to be given to keeping the area dry. Make sure that you are drying between any folds. It is also okay to use a hair dryer if needed.

MENSTRUAL HYGIENE

Special attention should be given to hygiene habits during your menstrual cycle. We all likely experienced "the lecture" around fifth grade when they separated the girls from the boys. I have no idea what the boys talked about. But for us girls, there was a discussion around starting your menstrual cycle and proper hygiene. From what I recall, we were only to use pads and bathe daily. Needless to say, the meeting left much to be desired about basic upkeep with menses. Without disclosing my age, fifth grade for me was many years ago. In speaking with my teenage niece, not much has changed. So, let's talk about the items that may not have been discussed in elementary school.

It is perfectly okay to use sanitary napkins with menses. The pads should be changed every time you go to the restroom or at least every three to four hours. The pads should be changed prior to bedtime and first thing in the morning. If possible, wash twice a day. It is perfectly okay to take a bath with menses.

Some women do not like the pubic hairs coated with blood. Removal of the blood can become difficult with showering. An easy solution to this problem is taking a bath, trimming the pubic hairs, or using tampons. Tampons may also be a solution for women who develop vulvar irritation from the sanitary napkins, or for female athletes. And yes, tampons can be used in women who are virgins. Tampons should be changed every four to eight hours. It is okay to use tampons at bedtime. The tampon should be changed prior to bedtime and first thing in the morning. Do not leave a tampon inside of you for longer than eight hours. The fear of prolonged use of tampons has always been toxic shock syndrome (TTS). The great news is that the length of time that the tampon is in place does not increase your risk of TTS. TTS is caused by bacteria. The association of TTS with tampons came with high absorbency tampons, which are no longer on the market.

Tampon selection can be an important determinant of your overall experience. Applicators may be cardboard or plastic. In general, women prefer one over the other for personal reasons. There is not a superior applicator. My personal preference is the plastic applicator. The tampon's level of absorbency may affect comfort level. For example, using a super absorbent tampon for mild vaginal bleeding may lead to vaginal dryness and irritation. Please choose an absorbency level that is consistent with your menstrual flow.

SEVEN CARDINAL SINS TO THE PRIVATE FACE

Over the years, counseling my patients about good, basic, and healthy vulvar and vaginal habits has been quite interesting. Often, both the teenage patient and her mother are unaware of how some common, daily habits can have negative effects on the Private Face. Because of this, I'm always sharing tips with my patients and parents about keeping our precious area safe. I call my tips the "Seven Cardinal Sins to the Private Face." These are tips that are easy to remember and therefore easy to share with others. As the old saying goes, "When we know better, we do better."

1) Commando in Jeans

Jeans are made of abrasive material. This will definitely increase the friction with the vulva, causing increased heat, moisture, sweating and trauma to the skin. This material is not very absorbable, which will exacerbate the problem. To add insult to injury, there is the seam of the jeans. It is easy to imagine the trauma it can cause.

2) Shaving without Shave Gel

The shave gel not only softens the hair, but it also hydrates the skin. This two-step process decreases the risk of ingrown hairs and trauma to the skin itself.

3) Prolonged Wearing of Swimsuit Bottoms

Wet swimsuit bottoms create a warm, moist area for bacteria and fungus to grow. Remove the swim bottoms when you get out of the water. Always bring dry cotton underwear and a dry pair of shorts or pants – or even a skirt – to wear after swimming.

4) Incomplete Drying of the Private Face

Even though your body is clean when you're done bathing, incomplete drying still creates the same setup as Number 3.

5) Using Community Razors on the Private Face

I cannot say it enough. Use a special razor for your special area. Using the same razor for your underarms and legs as you do on the vulva will increase your risk for bacterial spread.

6) Using a Dull Razor on the Private Face

A dull razor increases your risk for ingrown hairs. If you are using a disposable razor, the rule is "three and out," which means you can use the razor three times before replacement.

7) Ignoring the Private Face

The most disrespectful thing a woman can do to her Private Face is ignore it. Early recognition and treatment of multiple skin conditions can prevent chronic complications.

CHAPTER 13

BEAUTY BELOW MAINTENANCE REGIMENS

The Private Face deserves to be pampered. The vulva is more sensitive to injury than the public face, yet we give it less attention. We seldom consider the possibility of a vulvar medical condition. It is from this sacred area that life enters the world. For that reason alone, we should do more to maintain a healthy Private Face. I am offering you simple grooming routines to help you achieve and maintain healthy vulvar skin. Even though you are now aware of all the risks with specific grooming techniques, I will give you formulas based on your grooming preferences. I hope this book has empowered you to make healthy choices about grooming preferences.

In reference to grooming techniques, a woman's garden is divided into three categories. A full garden represents a woman with 50 percent or more of her pubic hairs. An arid garden has less than 50 percent of pubic hairs. The arid garden ranges from removal of the hairs of the bikini line to removal of all the hair of the external genitalia. Women who are postmenopausal, regardless of if they remove their hairs or not, have a mature garden. Whether you have a full garden (are unshaved), arid garden (shaved), or mature garden (postmenopausal), these grooming regimens should guide you toward better beauty practices for your Private Face.

BEAUTY BELOW GARDEN TOOLS

Trimming Scissors: Make sure that the tips are dull.

Comb: The comb should be small and thin toothed.

Shower glove: Make sure that the glove has an exfoliating and soft side. Again, the exfoliating side should only be used where there is hair. Avoid using the exfoliating side near the entry of the vagina.

THE FULL GARDEN SKINCARE

This vulvar skin regimen is for women who prefer their pubic hairs in the natural state. Even though many women choose to remove their pubic hairs, there is absolutely nothing wrong with keeping yours. Women with a full garden have the most significant potential for healthy, vulvar skin.

1) Wash daily with a mild soap or water.

As discussed earlier, it is your choice if you would like to use a mild soap or water. The key is removing residual discharge, sebum produced by the hair follicles, or other products such as semen that can become trapped in the labial folds or pubic hairs. Only use the soft side of a shower glove on the non-hairy areas.

2) Use a thin tooth comb on the Private Face hairs while bathing.

213

It is common for pubic hairs to become tangled. The thin comb serves two purposes. First, it is your detangler. Secondly – and most importantly – the comb functions as your exfoliator. As you gently move the comb through your hairs, the tips of the comb help remove dead skin cells.

3) Apply a dry oil hair (or beard) softener at least three times per week after bathing.

Daily washing can strip the pubic hairs of their natural oils. The dry hair oil serves as your leave-in conditioner. While helping to balance the natural oils of your garden, it also softens the hair follicles. The softening of the hair follicles will help to prevent ingrown hairs.

4) Trim excess hairs at least twice a month.

When the garden is very thick or "overgrown," women can experience excess sweating. Trimming the garden will aid in the prevention of excess sweating. Let's not forget that earlier in the book, you learned that your pubic hairs help to absorb sweat. That statement is true. But too much of anything can cause some problems. Simple trimming should be considered for all women with a full garden. Trimming the garden also alleviates the trapping of menstrual blood within the pubic hairs.

THE ARID GARDEN SKINCARE

If your preference is for partial or complete removal of pubic hairs, this routine is for you. Women who only remove bikini hairs may incorporate both the full and arid garden hygiene regimens. Before deciding to remove your pubic hairs, please review the hair removal risks discussed earlier in this book. Understanding the risks associated with removing the Private Face strands is the initial step to achieving and maintaining healthy vulvar skin. It is essential to have a beauty regimen that is specific to your grooming preference. The following is a recommended Private Face hygiene routine for those who choose to remove pubic hairs via shaving, waxing, sugaring, laser, or electrolysis.

1) Wash daily with a mild soap.

If you choose to remove your pubic hairs, washing with only water is not an option. You have removed one of the body's natural defenses. There is therefore no hair to absorb the sweat or block the vulvar skin from potential irritants. Daily washing will help remove waste from our natural vaginal discharge, sweat, and external materials.

It is also important to wash with warm water before any hair removal procedure. A warm wash will remove dirt, open the pores, and make the hair softer before removal. Washing with warm water before shaving procedures will decrease infection risk, trauma to the skin, and ingrown hairs.

2) Daily moisturizer

Here, we are not talking about a moisturizer for the vagina. We are discussing a moisturizer for the outside skin, or vulva. The moisturizer will protect the skin from drying and chaffing. It will also protect us from external factors such as our clothing. Every woman who is removing the hair from down there should use a moisturizer. Pubic hair removal increases your risk for vulvar skin dryness. As discussed in Chapter 4, the sebum produced on the pubic hairs is a natural moisturizer of the hair and vulvar skin.

3) Weekly exfoliation

A shower glove is recommended with daily washing. The exfoliating side of the glove is one form of exfoliation. For women who choose to remove the pubic hairs, exfoliation must be more extensive in order to prevent ingrown hairs. A weekly gentle, chemical exfoliator is needed. Do not exfoliate on the day of any hair removal procedure. Some women, depending on hair removal techniques, should also avoid exfoliation the day *before* any hair removal procedures. Women with sensitive skin may be more prone to develop transient irritation of the skin. If skin irritation is already present prior to hair removal, further damage to the skin is likely to occur.

4) Skin toner after hair removal

After any form of hair removal, the use of a skin toner is necessary. The toner will help remove any residual products used to remove the hair. A warm wash will open the pores before hair removal, and toner will close the pores. The right toner also has anti-inflammatory properties. It will help prevent redness and irritation after your hair removal procedure. The toner also helps prepare the skin for your moisturizer. Always apply the toner before the moisturizer.

THE MATURE GARDEN SKINCARE

The mature garden references women who have reached menopause. Menopause occurs when a woman has been without a menstrual cycle for at least 12 months or has removed her ovaries. This means that she has not seen blood down there – not even spotting – for over one year. As with our public face, many changes occur with the Private Face over time. The natural transition of the Private Face is detailed earlier in the book. Many changes occur because of the loss of estrogen during menopause. The postmenopausal beauty-below regimen promotes health and anti-aging.

1) Wash daily with a mild soap.

As we age, the hair of the Private Face becomes thinner and scant. Because of less hair, a mild wash as opposed to water should be used. The exfoliation side of the shower glove should only be used on the mons pubis.

2) Use a comb while bathing.

If hair is still present, the use of a thin, dulled tooth comb will aid in detangling and exfoliation.

3) Daily anti-aging serum with hyaluronic acid.

For those with sparse hairs, anti-aging serum should be used. The serum will help to keep the skin supple in appearance and decrease fine lines or wrinkles.

4) Daily moisturizer on the vulva.

A daily moisturizer is imperative with the mature garden. Keeping the skin moisturized will help prevent wrinkles of the Private Face.

5) A vaginal moisturizer twice a week.

If there is even a small amount of vaginal dryness, a daily moisturizer should be used. Here, we are talking about a moisturizer that is specifically for the vagina. This may not be the same moisturizer that you will use on the vulva. Remember that the outside of the Private Face is treated differently than the inside. Please consult with your healthcare provider prior to placing any products inside of your vagina. The goal of the daily application of a moisturizer is to prevent extensive vaginal dryness, which can lead to irritation, microtears and pain with intercourse. A moisturizer is different than a lubricant. As stated before, a moisturizer is used to prevent or treat vaginal dryness. A lubricant is used to aid with sex.

THE BUMP STOPPER SKINCARE

Special care should be given to women who suffer with recurrent, extensive bumps of the Private Face. A proactive approach will help women to either prevent or decrease the recurrence or extent of disease. Shaving with a razor is not recommended in this subset of women. If you are removing your pubic hairs by other methods, please review the recommendations under the Arid Garden.

1) Wash daily with a mild soap.

Due to the increased risk of infection, it is imperative to wash daily. The shower glove will aid in exfoliation.

2) Use a comb with bathing.

A dull, single tooth comb will detangle pubic hairs and provide some removal of dead skin cells.

3) Use a hair oil three times a week.

A dry hair oil will soften the hairs. The softening of curly, coarse hair will decrease the hairs' ability to pierce the skin and create an ingrown hair.

4) Exfoliate weekly.

With pseudo-folliculitis barbae, exfoliation is imperative to the management of this disease. The removal of dead skin cells will help dislodge and prevent ingrown hairs.

5) Vaniqa (Eflornithine HCL 13.9%) Rx twice a day

This is a prescription-strength medication which decreases the rate of hair growth. The effects of this medication are generally noted after about one to two months of use.

6) Vitamin A – topical

Vitamin A helps to reduce skin plugging and buildup of dead skin cells. There is a prescription strength medication called Retin-A. Talk to your doctor about using Vitamin A in pregnancy or while attempting pregnancy. There are now over-the-counter products that contain Vitamin A. Stop Vitamin A application at least 72 hours prior to any hair removal procedures. You can restart the Vitamin A 48 hours after the procedure. Do not exfoliate and use Vitamin A on the same day.

CHAPTER 14

PRODUCT SELECTION GUIDE

Throughout this book you have learned about various products that can maintain and enhance the Private Face. If you are anything like me, you have stood in the drug store for a ridiculous length of time trying to determine the best product to use on your public face, or even body. You have asked yourself about the significance of a cream being plant-based or all-natural. What does all this mean? How do I know which product is best for me? This chapter will give you a framework to product selection by answering common, frequently asked questions. It is important to note that except for color additives, the law does not require FDA premarket approval for cosmetic products and ingredients.

SHOULD I ONLY USE PRODUCTS THAT ARE HYPOALLERGENIC?

The FDA refers to "hypoallergenic" as products that manufacturers claim produce fewer allergic reactions than other cosmetic products.[13] However, there are no standards or definitions that products must meet in order to put "hypoallergenic" on the label. The manufacturer does not have to prove that the product will not cause a reaction. Additionally, it is impossible to guarantee that a product will *never* cause an allergic reaction. Therefore, do not allow the claim "hypoallergenic" to influence your decision in purchasing a skincare product. As with all new products, test it on a small area of the skin prior to general use.

---

[13]   https://www.fda.gov/cosmetics/labeling-claims/hypoallergenic-cosmetics/index.htm

WHAT IS THE DIFFERENCE BETWEEN NATURAL AND ORGANIC?

The claim that a product is natural simply means that it contains ingredients that come from natural sources. If the main ingredient is plant-based, a natural product may still contain preservatives or chemicals. "Organic" implies that the product contains naturally sourced ingredients produced without chemicals or pesticides. Organic products are not FDA-regulated. However, the National Organic Program under the USDA regulates and certifies organic products. Cosmetic products labeled as "organic" must comply with both USDA regulations for the organic claim and FDA requirements for labeling and safety. The overall perceived benefits of organic products are that they are free from ingredients that are known to have adverse effects on the human body. Always remember that an ingredient's source **does not** determine its safety.

WHAT IS PH BALANCED ALL ABOUT?

PH stands for potential of hydrogen, or power of hydrogen. It measures the activity of hydrogen ions in a watery solution. PH is used to measure the acidity or basicity of a solution. The pH runs from 0-14. High pH means that the solution is basic. A low pH means that the solution is acidic. A pH of 7 is considered neutral. The skin on any part of the body is most effective when at its ideal pH level. The pH balance is especially important in the vulvar/vaginal area. If the pH is too basic, it will become dry, aged, and prone to infection. If the pH is acidic, the skin can become red, inflamed, and itchy. PH imbalance can be caused by diet, hormones, and environmental stressors such as soaps. In most cases, the pH of a product is not listed. Sometimes, the quoted pH is inaccurate. To determine the pH of your beauty products, consider using pH strips or litmus papers. When it comes to the care down there, make sure that your cleansers, moisturizers, and such do not exceed a pH of 6. Consider using a water softener or shower head filter. The best water for skin pH is soft, non-alkaline, and with a low mineral count. Always wash with lukewarm water. Hot water can disrupt the pH and damage the skin.

IS FRAGRANCE-FREE RIGHT FOR ME?

The term "fragrance free" implies that no extra fragrance is added to change the product's naturally occurring aroma. Keep in mind that fragrance-free products can still contain fragrance compounds. Fragrant ingredients can be in the original formula. "Unscented" products may contain a masking fragrance. There is no legal definition or FDA regulation for the claims of "unscented" or "fragrance free." The concern for fragrances is that some people can have a skin reaction to the fragrance or negative respiratory symptoms. However, fewer than 10 percent of people with skin problems are allergic to fragrance. It is important to note that there are both synthetic and natural fragrances. Some of the bad actors to avoid are amyl cinnamal, benzoyl alcohol, and cinnamyl alcohol. Check out the European Commission's Scientific Committee on Consumer Safety for a list of 26 chemicals to avoid. Unless you have a known sensitivity to any fragrance, there is no need to be fragrance free. [14] Look for high-quality natural fragrances such as vanilla, cucumber, mango, aloe vera, or coconut. An important fact to note is that manufacturers are not required to list the ingredients of their fragrances. Some, however, will provide more details within their advertising and packaging.

---

[14]

https://ec.europa.eu/health/scientific_committees/opinions_layman/perfume-allergies/en/index.htm

WHAT IS A PARABEN?

Within the health and beauty industry, you will see many advertisements for paraben-free products. What does that mean? Why are parabens bad for me? Parabens are a group of mostly synthetic chemicals that act as a preservative in many cosmetics products. They allow the products to have a longer shelf life by preventing the growth of bacteria and fungus. Parabens are often found in shampoos, soaps, and skincare products. They can mimic the estrogen hormone. Some feel that the chronic use of parabens in beauty products can lead to an increase of parabens in breast tissue, which will increase human breast cancer cells. A direct link of parabens to breast cancer has not been established. The FDA and the American Cancer Society recognize parabens as safe for use in consumer products.[15] If you are concerned about a

---

[15] https://www.cdc.gov/biomonitoring/Paragens_FactSheet.html

possible link to breast cancer, look for names such as methylparaben, ethylparaben, propylparaben, and similar terms. Remember that paraben-free *does not* mean that the product is chemical-free. The product may contain another preservative with unknown risks. Look for natural preservative options such as rosemary extract or grapefruit seed extract.

IS SULFATE SOMETHING I SHOULD HATE?

A sulfate is a salt that is produced from petroleum or plant sources such as coconut oil and palm oil. The most common sulfates are sodium lauryl sulfate and sodium laureth sulfate. They create the lather in cleaning products, which gives a stronger impression of cleaning power. Sulfates act as a surfactant, which allows the product to spread easily and lift water, dirt, and oils from the hair and skin. Sulfates do not cause cancer, infertility, or developmental delays. Their biggest risk is irritation to the skin, eyes, or lungs. They may also cause drying of the hair by removing too much of the natural oils. This is more of an issue when you are considering which shampoo to use. However, those with rosacea or sensitive skin may choose to use a sulfate-free wash. A sulfate-free wash will be more hydrating and lack the foam or lather. The lather is not a necessary component to clean skin. Some natural alternatives to sulfates are solid or oil-based soaps. Some people avoid sulfates due to environmental concerns. The sulfates from petroleum are associated with climate change and greenhouse gases. For example, palm oil comes from palm tree plantations that are thought to contribute to the destruction of the rainforest.

IS SILICONE BAD FOR MY SKIN?

Silicone is a semi-liquid substance made from silica. Sand is mainly made of silica, for example. In order to become silicone, silica has to undergo an aggressive chemical process. Common names for silicone are dimethicone, cyclomethicone, and cyclohexasiloxane. Silicone functions as a barrier coating on skin that is resistant to water and air.

In the medical world, silicone helps to heal wounds and resolve scarring. In the cosmetic world, silicone allows the skin to appear plump and smooth, without any true health benefit. The downside to silicone is that it doesn't rinse away easily. The barrier that it creates can trap oil, dirt, and dead skin cells. For those who are acne-prone, the use of silicone on the skin can make acne worse. For everyone else, it is not necessary to include or eliminate silicone from your products. In addition, silicone is not eco-friendly. It is known to contribute to the buildup of sludge in the ocean and waterways.

WHAT ARE PHTHALATES?

Phthalates are a group of plastic enhancers that are used in cosmetics to mask unpleasant odors. Some people believe that phthalates can disrupt female hormones, exacerbate asthma, and cause neurodevelopmental disorders in children. These claims have not been proven. The CDC states that the effects of phthalates are unknown.[16] More research is needed prior to claiming that phthalates can be harmful to human health.

---

[16] https://www.cdc.gov/biomonitoring/Phthalates_FactSheet.html

PHASE 4: OWN THE PRIVATE FACE

CONCLUSION

There is no such thing as a perfect Private Face. However, your Private Face was made perfectly for you. Within this book you have been given the knowledge to maintain the health of the vulva and vagina. Understanding the skin below the waist – and having the confidence to talk about it – will improve overall wellness.

You now have the enhanced ability to prevent vulvar skin conditions and to recognize diseased states early enough to decrease the chances of long-term or permanent damage. I hope this book supports the appreciation of vulvas in all their various shapes, sizes, and colors. I also hope, upon the completion of this book, that you will be empowered to include the maintenance of healthy vulvar skin in your wellness routine.

As we remove the shame associated with the vulva and vagina, let's be mindful to avoid shaming those who choose to explore aesthetics for the Private Face. No one shames a woman for dyeing the hair upon her head or applying lipstick before leaving her residence. It is each woman's own prerogative in her choices for the appearance of her Private Face, too. My resolve is to keep each woman and her Private Face as healthy as possible while also respecting her aesthetic preferences.

In the next book, we will cover the last phase of the Beauty Below Formula: OWNing your Private Face. I look forward to teaching you how to optimize the skincare of the vulva and the effectiveness of the vagina. I am excited to ride along on your journey to maximizing the Beauty Below. Finally, skincare products, specifically customized for intimate wellness and beauty for dark skin, are available at www.BeautyBelowMD.com.

APPENDIX

SUPPORT GROUPS FOR VARIOUS CONDITIONS OF THE PRIVATE FACE

Vulvodynia

The National Vulvodynia Association

www.nva.org

Vaginismus

Vaginismus Support Group

www.mazewomenshealth.com/forums/forum/vaginismus/

Vaginismus

Women's Therapy Center

https://www.womentc.com/conditions-and-

treatments/penetration-pain-disorders/vaginismus/vaginismus-a-private-pain-support-group/

Hidradenitis Supprativa

Hope for HS

www.hopeforhs.org

Vaginal Cancer

Cancer Care

www.cancercare.org/support_groups/176-

living_with_cancer_gynecologic_cancers_patient_support_

group

Herpes

American Sexual Health Association

www.ashasexualhealth.org/herpes-support-groups/

Vulvar Cancer

Smart Patients

https://www.smartpatients.com/communities/vulvar-cancer

Lichen Sclerosus

Smart Patients

www.smartpatients.com/communities/vulvar-cancer

Lichen Sclerosus

https://lichensclerosuspodcast.com/do-you-need-a-support-group/

About the Author

Dr. Cynthia Wesley is a board-certified OBGYN who has dedicated more than twenty years to educating women on the best practices for ultimate vulvar/vaginal wellness, as well as on conditions that affect its viability. She completed her undergraduate degree, medical school, and residency training in Obstetrics and Gynecology at West Virginia University. She uses her passion and expertise to excel as a national speaker, a vulvar skin specialist, and the Founder and CEO of Beauty Below, a product line focused on intimate wellness and beauty for dark skin. She is a contributing author of *Navigating a Triple Pandemic.* Affectionately and respectfully known as "Dr. Cyn," Dr. Wesley resides in North Carolina with her daughter.

Learn more at www.BeautyBelowMD.com

Made in the USA
Columbia, SC
02 November 2021